Praise for *Chakra Wisc*

C000224685

"This book is one of few that could rightly
shifting'—in more than one sense of the word. ... In *Chakra Wisaom*,
Trish O'Sullivan lucidly provides practical techniques for purifying
the mind and forging a robust mind-body connection. As a profes-
sor of Ayurveda and physician for more than thirty years, I am ac-
customed to viewing the mind through the filter of ancient Indian
concepts: *buddhi, manas, aha kara,* and *samskara. Chakra Wisdom's*
clear and eloquent language describes how to translate these concepts
into actions that promote healing; I also believe these same techniques
could, for some individuals, help create a transformation of human
consciousness itself. *Chakra Wisdom* is an invitation to insight, to
true identity, to wholeness. Everyone who uses these exercises can
expect to be awakened progressively to various hitherto unseen subtle
dimensions of the human being."

—Scott Gerson, MD, PhD, Medical Director of the Jupiter Medical
Center Department of Integrative Medicine, Division of Education and
Research, and Medical Director of the Gerson Institute of Ayurvedic
Medicine

CHAKRA
WISDOM

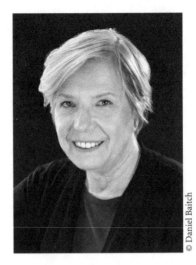

© Daniel Baitch

About the Author

Trish O'Sullivan (New York) is a licensed clinical social worker, a senior dharma teacher in the Kwan Um School of Zen, and a certified yoga teacher. In addition to her private psychotherapy practice, she conducts Traya technique trainings for individuals, psychotherapists, and yoga therapy practitioners. Trish has published articles in *The Journal of Psychology and Religion* and *The Encyclopedia of Psychology and Religion*.

TRISH O'SULLIVAN

CHAKRA WISDOM

HEALING NEGATIVE THOUGHTS,
FEELINGS, AND BELIEFS WITH MEDITATION,
YOGA, AND THE TRAYA PROCESS

Llewellyn Publications
Woodbury, Minnesota

FIRST EDITION
First Printing, 2018

Cover design by Kristi Carlson
Editing by Brian R. Erdrich
Interior illustrations by Mary Ann Zapalac

Llewellyn Publications is a registered trademark of Llewellyn Worldwide Ltd.

Library of Congress Cataloging-in-Publication Data (Pending)
ISBN: 978-0-7387-5743-8

Llewellyn Worldwide Ltd. does not participate in, endorse, or have any authority or responsibility concerning private business transactions between our authors and the public.
   All mail addressed to the author is forwarded but the publisher cannot, unless specifically instructed by the author, give out an address or phone number.
   Any internet references contained in this work are current at publication time, but the publisher cannot guarantee that a specific location will continue to be maintained. Please refer to the publisher's website for links to authors' websites and other sources.

Llewellyn Publications
A Division of Llewellyn Worldwide Ltd.
2143 Wooddale Drive
Woodbury, MN 55125-2989
www.llewellyn.com

Printed in the United States of America

This book is dedicated to my spiritual teachers in gratitude for their wisdom, generosity, and boundless patience
Elsie Becherer (in memoriam)
Zen Master Wu Kwang (Richard Shrobe)

Disclaimer

Contents

List of Exercises

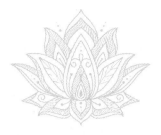

INTRODUCTION

For most of human history, people practiced the religion they were born into. Today we have an abundance of choice in both the material and spiritual marketplaces, and many pick and choose practices from different spiritual paths. Meditation and yoga, once considered esoteric practices in the West, have seeped into the mainstream. Once a regular practice is established, the benefits are so evident that it is hard to imagine life without either of these. It is my great fortune to be able to offer a third practice that both supports and is supported by meditation and yoga.

Traya means "three" in Sanskrit and the practice I have developed is so named because it is a mind, body, and spirit practice that provides a new way of engaging with and healing the chakras. The development of Traya is the result of a long journey involving good fortune, dedication, growth, and transformation.

How the Traya Process Came About

I was fortunate to find special teachers on my journey. In the late 1970s, I found Elsie, who taught yoga before it was widespread in New York City. She introduced me to many gurus, geshes, and masters from a variety of traditions who she met through her position at a bookstore. She lent me books and introduced me to some of these esteemed teachers, and I became taken with Eastern spirituality, especially Buddhism. I later found a home in the Kwan Um School of Zen and—in honor of my first teacher, Elsie, who had passed on—I continued my yoga practice and eventually became certified to teach yoga.

In spite of all of this involvement with Eastern spirituality, I hadn't had any exposure to the chakras beyond reading about them in tantric and new age books. Then by serendipity I met Nancy Rosanoff, who taught intuitive development, and I took some of her classes. I learned several techniques for engaging with the chakras and accessing information, most notably a unique technique (somewhat like a shamanic journey) for cleansing them of toxic psychic energy. I continued to use these techniques on myself and I noticed that my thinking began to change and I became more positive. I modified the techniques I learned from Nancy and established a daily practice. I discovered that my significant fears decreased if I focused on a particular chakra in a mindful way and continued to clear it. My thoughts became more positive, my confidence and self-esteem increased, and many more benefits appeared and stayed. My mind was changing!

I continued to search through both Western and Eastern books, looking for information on or similar to this process, but was never able to find anything akin to what I was finding on my own. Although I was frustrated at the time, now I see that this lack of outside information turned out to be a great boon. It forced me to do the work myself and, in the process, I learned that the capacity for self-healing is innate within each of us. The chakras become accessible and understandable. They teach us. We can even put aside whatever information about the chakras we have been exposed to, as we don't need to know anything about a chakra in order to work with it. In fact, we may get in our own way if we have too many preconceived ideas.

At some point in my development of Traya, I crossed a threshold. I discovered that I was being led by a force within that was guiding me and leading me toward wholeness—my Inner Teacher. I was steadfast in my exploration, and as I progressed I was able to learn more and more. The truth of the interconnectedness of the chakras, mind, body, and spirit became apparent. Different facets and deeper and subtler layers of meaning were revealed and I felt as though I was bathing in wisdom. At first I felt as though I was teasing out the secrets of the mind, but then the mind began to guide the whole process and I felt as though I was following instead of leading. I felt embraced by my higher self and by the universe. I was a participant in my own metamorphosis, attaining intimacy with my own mind.

I began to work with others and gained similar results. The common patterns I saw from person to person revealed what types of experiences produced negative issues in each particular chakra. It also showed the associated problematic thoughts, feelings, and behaviors. While the main function of many of the seven primary chakras are well-established, I learned that each chakra had many previously unknown attributes. I found smaller chakras between the seven major chakras, and their important functions and effects became clear.

I wanted to see how the Traya techniques could be integrated with traditional psychotherapy, so I went back to school and eventually obtained my license as a psychotherapist. I found that the Traya techniques fit nicely into the psychotherapeutic setting, allowing a therapist to combine Western and Eastern techniques and approaches. At the same time, I continued doing workshops and teaching people Traya techniques to use on their own.

Why Practice Traya?

This book can help you to develop a working relationship with the subtle body and your Inner Teacher. Many who experience the insights and benefits of Traya express the same regret: "I wish that I had known about these techniques earlier in my life." My answer to them has been, "Most people never have this opportunity." I am astonished by my good fortune in being led to develop Traya and am both humbled and honored to be able to offer it to you.

There is a growing phenomenon in which Eastern spiritual practices spill over into the Western psychotherapy field. One need only google the term "mindfulness" to find several Western therapies that use the Buddhist mindfulness practice to cope with afflictive thoughts and emotions. On the other hand, there is also the "spiritual bypass," a termed coined by John Welwood that refers to the use of spirituality to avoid unpleasant emotions and unresolved psychological issues. People are seeking relief from negative thoughts and feelings in spirituality, and at the same time, spiritual practices such as mindfulness and meditation are borrowed by the field of psychotherapy. Traya has elements of Buddhist and yoga psychology and like those practices can be approached from a secular perspective, but is essentially a spiritual practice. Since Traya is grounded in both Eastern and Western worlds, this is a perfect time for the practice to be introduced to a wider audience.

Modern psychology teaches that the evolutionary process has left us with a mind in conflict with itself. It teaches that the mind speaks through its symptoms and neuroses and can be managed but not fully healed. Traya expands both the quality and quantity of interaction with the mind by allowing for a direct connection to the deep mind by becoming mindful of the subtle body. We find that what is going on there is not what we thought. Thus, it establishes a completely new paradigm.

The mind is energy, and until we meet it on an energetic level, we cannot really change it. The most wondrous thing we find is that the mind wants to be detoxified and assists us in the process. The mind is not our enemy after all. Traya is an organic process available to all of us that cleanses the mind of negativity. When I first encountered these techniques, I used them as an adjunct to the therapy I was already in. That worked well until my intense dedication to this practice and the support from my Inner Teacher that I had come to trust over time gave me the sense that I was standing on the shoulders of the universe. I had outgrown my need to work with someone else. You will see in chapter 5 on the stages of change that Traya leads to a reversal of the tendency to look outside for answers.

Growing Spiritually

Even though I draw on a background based in Eastern traditions and perspective, it's OK if you don't resonate with this perspective. Your own individual spiritual connection and practice is what will enable you to complete the entire process of change outlined in this book.

There are questions lying deep within that call out to be both asked and answered. In my in-depth exploration of the chakras, I found not only psychological truths but also spiritual truths. I found how to diminish that sense of separateness we feel from our higher self, others, and spirit. In fact, Traya supports every aspect of life: emotional, mental, physical, and spiritual.

Meditation and yoga nourish us, deepen our spiritual connection, and allow us to enter the stream. Traya provides yet another level of engagement with ourselves that we are currently unaware of. All three practices reinforce one another, supporting what I call the "Lotus of Full Potential," which blooms organically and completely within us.

Understanding the Book Format and Style

As you move through the book, there are some formatting styles that will be helpful for you to be aware of. Firstly, quoted material that is surfaced directly from a chakra and spoken by a client in a Traya session is italicized in order to distinguish it from other comments and discussions. This is not to be confused with the introduction of a new Sanskrit or foreign word, which, in publication, is traditionally italicized when first mentioned.

Traya has roots in the tantric world of medieval India that recognized the subtle body and the chakra system. To honor that origin, I keep the Sanskrit terms for each of the primary chakras and provide additional Sanskrit names for the new subsystem of chakras (the secondary chakras) that I encountered while working with my clients.

To ensure ease of understanding for those who are new to the Sanskrit chakra names, I will most often refer to the seven primary chakras by their location, e.g., the heart chakra, the throat chakra, etc. To more readily distinguish the seven secondary chakras, I refer to them by their function, e.g., the imagination chakra, the self-esteem chakra, etc. There were other useful terms that I borrowed from the Sanskrit, such as *samskaras* for mind imprints. It is close enough in meaning to be applicable. Traya is, I believe, appropriately wrapped in the fabric of yoga psychology while, at the same time, completely new.

The book is presented in two parts. In part 1 you will learn about the subtle body and ways to connect with it (including meditation and yoga) as well as how negativity forms in the mind and the Traya approach to healing it. Part 2 provides a comprehensive discussion of each chakra (including the "new" secondaries) with all their attributes listed and explained. Each of these chapters include client examples of material surfaced from each chakra demonstrating the types of situations that impact them. Clients are disguised along with some of the minor details of their experiences for confidentiality purposes. There is a lot of information and if you are anxious to get working on a chakra, you can skip some of this material and come back to it later. There are many exercises throughout the book to help you along your way.

I offer this information to you. I hope that you approach it with openness, excitement, respect, diligence, and patience so that you may become completely human and bloom the Lotus of Full Potential within you.

Part 1

THE MIND AND THE
TRAYA PROCESS

This section provides an overview of the subtle body, its relationship to the mind, and the Traya approach to healing the mind. Central to this system are the *chakras*, which are psychospiritual energy centers in the body that produce various mind functions and states of mind.

The first chapter outlines a new perspective on the mind and how it incorporates negativity and creates a "pain body." The second chapter outlines the structure of the subtle body and clarifies the relationship between the mind and the subtle body chakras.

The following chapters provide information on working directly with the chakras and, most importantly and uniquely to this book, completely new techniques for diagnosing the health of a chakra, lifting negativity from the mind, and the stages of change in healing the pain body. In chapter 4 there is a discussion of the relationship between meditation and yoga and the subtle body, how these practices support the Traya healing process, and vice versa. Chapter 5 outlines the Traya process of change, growth, and transformation.

In part 2 you will delve deeper into the individual chakras, understanding their functions and attributes, and the type of memories that impact them. The exercises related to each chakra will help you put the Traya techniques into practice. If you would like to skip ahead and dive into the specific chakra work, read chapter 3 and then move on to part 2.

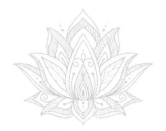

Chapter 1

A NEW PERSPECTIVE ON THE MIND
(or How the Mind Really Works)

The term "mind" is understood differently by various theorists and schools of thought. My Zen and yoga studies and intimate work with the chakras have revealed a simple yet profound mind structure. Viewing the mind from this perspective helps to clarify the relationship between the mind and the subtle body chakras.

Two Levels of Mind

When we think about the mind, we usually think of the part of us that observes, thinks, plans, remembers, and analyzes. We know that there is another part of the mind that is not readily accessible to this conscious mind, and this other part has been given different labels—the unconscious, preconscious, subconscious, instinctual, intuitive, and subliminal mind. Less confusing and more meaningful, as we will see, is to refer to the conscious mind as the "surface mind" and all other parts of the mind as the "deep mind."

"Deep mind" is a fitting term because while it is generally not directly accessible to the surface mind, it is certainly not unconscious or unaware. In fact, it is supremely conscious of every nuance of every experience even if the surface mind is not. It never misses anything and actively attempts to communicate with and guide us. It is not just a repository for storing memories but an active force always attempting to move us forward in our personal evolution.

Other than when we are sleeping, our mind operates on these two levels simultaneously. The surface mind needs to be free to do its unique job so there is a "veil" of unawareness that allows the surface mind to operate without being overwhelmed by input from the deep mind. This veil is not impermeable—it does not screen out all input from the deep mind but serves to screen out enough to keep the focus primarily in the surface mind.

Let's look at an example that illustrates this basic separation: A colleague calls me to make a lunch date to discuss something very important and we are focusing on where and when to meet—I need my surface mind attention to find the name and location of the restaurant and we agree on the time and place. The deep mind is both registering the interaction and providing information as to how I feel about the interaction. Suppose this colleague has a history of making dates and then sometimes canceling at the last minute. I don't feel right about making another date with him, but I am thrown off by the phrase "something very important." I feel a constriction in the pit of my stomach and some fear about having to confront this person about past behavior if I don't consent to the lunch. I go over the pros and cons. Should I call him back and what would I say?

The part of the mind that is thinking this through is the surface mind and the part that signals caution and fear is the deep mind. While we are making the date, we may not be so aware of this discomfort as we are "in" the surface mind focusing on time and place. The surface mind, while reviewing pros and cons, is not focused on the energy in the deep mind that is being stimulated by this interaction. For example, if we harbor a fear of confrontation, fear energy will be activated.

We can see that this perspective on the mind is, actually, the opposite of how we have traditionally viewed the mind—the "conscious mind" or surface mind has limited awareness and the unconscious or deep mind is aware of everything all the time—limitless. The deep mind attempts to communicate with the surface mind and make it more aware through feelings and thoughts generated by the dynamics of energy centers located at points along the axis of the spine called chakras.

The next chapter further explains and maps this system. Now let's look at how chakra dynamics influence both the surface and the deep mind.

Chakras and the Mind

I often use the analogy of a computer to help illustrate the relationship of the chakras and the mind. A computer needs three things to function: hardware, software, and power (electricity). The mind has these same three components: the brain (hardware), the chakras (software), and *prana* (power), also known as subtle energy. Each chakra energizes and influences a part of the mind by producing a unique consciousness that governs how we think about and experience both our inner and outer worlds. How well each chakra performs is dependent on the quality and quantity of prana available to that chakra. Thus the mind extends well beyond our brains.

All activity is an expression of subtle energy in the mind and body. When we interact with our environment and the people in it, there is an energetic interchange, and every experience has an energetic imprint associated with it. These imprints remain in the chakras in the form of memories and include aspects of the experience that didn't register in the surface mind at the time. Therefore, in this book, the word "memory" refers to all material surfaced from either the surface or deep mind. Traya completes the memory by bringing to consciousness aspects that didn't register in the surface mind at the time of the incident.

For example, Carolyn's mother was not around much, but Carolyn remembers that at the age of four or five her mom taught her how to make her own scrambled eggs. She remembers how much she liked that attention her mother paid to her. While she remembers the incident well and fondly, she did not consciously register the subliminal message—"Take care of yourself, I am not going to take care of you forever"—as she was focused on getting the attention she craved during the lesson. The deep mind did register that message as it is aligned with truth, and the truth was that the mother was neglectful, so a negative memory imprint or wound formed. It is quite common for people to say when discussing a highlighted memory imprint, "Oh, I didn't realize that," or, "I never thought of it that way."

Gloria recently said to me, "If you had asked me before starting this work if I was a lonely child, I would have said no. Now I see that I was."

In yoga psychology, experience residues are termed *samskaras*. Collections of similarly themed samskaras, such as a variety of experiences related to a lack of choice, for example, are called *vasanas*. Before we look at how to work with these samskaras and vasanas, let's make sure we understand how they form.

Negative samskaras disrupt the flow of prana and produce tendencies counter to the function of the chakra. Positive samskaras enhance the prana and support the function of the chakra. In this book, the term "samskara" will most often refer to a negative imprint. Positive ones will be so identified. Again, using the analogy of the chakras as computer programs, a negative samskara is like a virus preventing a program from functioning as it was designed.

In the example of Carolyn's cooking lesson, a samskara formed in her heart chakra (*anahata*), the chakra of connection and caring, when the deep mind registered her mother's neglect. Carolyn has a wounded heart chakra that can no longer provide a sense of confidence in people and her connection to them as this chakra was designed to provide. Instead she has an abiding sense of sadness and abandonment that will be stimulated at various times by events in her life, and she will feel this wound again and again. Her thoughts, feelings, relationships, and life will all be influenced by that simple experience. Of course, that incident was representative of a lack of involvement by her mother that was found in many of her other childhood memories.

This accumulation of samskaras, if not healed, will continue to grow over time. Her lack of connection energy will drive poor choices that will produce new samskaric experiences outside of the home and throughout her life. The original samskaras and their resulting shoots and branches together will form what Eckhart Tolle termed the "pain body."

The Pain Body

Eckart Tolle in *The Power of Now* describes this phenomenon well although he is not discussing the chakras specifically: "This accumulated pain is a negative energy field that occupies your body and mind. If you look on it as an invisible entity in its own right, you are getting quite close to the truth. It's the emotional pain body."[1] He goes on to say that this pain body "consists of trapped life-energy that has split off from your total energy field and has temporarily become autonomous."[2] This perspective helps us to understand that the accumulated samskaras are separate from us—they are entities with their own thoughts, feelings, and beliefs. When we experience negativity, it feels like it is a part of us, as it comes from within in the form of thoughts and feelings. But we wouldn't think of a virus as a part of a computer and we shouldn't think of negative thoughts or feelings as part of us either. We pick up samskaras from our environment just as we do biological viruses.

There is a Sanskrit term for negative states of mind—*kleshas*. Kleshas include destructive emotions such as anger and fear as well as other mind afflictions such as jealousy, distrust, greed, etc. Negative samskaras produce kleshas, and the accumulation of kleshas results in the pain body. When the pain body dominates the mind, there is suffering in both the internal and external worlds, as what is inside is created outside.

The mind is energy and everything that the mind creates is a form of energy. Thoughts are energy, feelings are energy, and states of mind are energy. I often refer to samskaric patterns in the chakras as "fear energy" or "sad energy." States of mind such as "disadvantaged," "victim," "outsider," etc., are all composed of energy, and when you take them apart or de-energize them with the Traya process, they disappear. So rather than try to convince someone not to feel a certain way, Traya

---

1. Eckart Tolle, *The Power of Now: A Guide to Spiritual Enlightenment* (Novato, CA: New World Library, 1999), 36.
2. Ibid., 39.

deals directly with the energy that is creating the state of mind and transforms it to positive, returning the mind to its innate positive state.

To reiterate, the chakras drive the dynamics of our lives, governing how we think, feel, and in large part, act. The past is never really the past as samskaric mind imprints operating in the deep mind influence the present and create the future.

Painful patterns too are rooted in the past, and if we don't uproot them, they continue to grow like weeds in our minds. Undigested wounds condition our expectations and responses, and more samskaras are accumulated by unwise or unwholesome decisions and actions. I saw this with John, a successful businessman who was working with me on his difficult marital relationship. We were exploring his heart chakra and the following came up:

…As a kid I felt that I was OK, but people around me were not.

He was referring to his family members who were dramatic and often in conflict. This memory came because his connection to his family was impacted by this conflict pattern and connection is the function of the heart chakra.

It suddenly dawned on him that this pattern was continuing to play out in his marriage and at work where he was often the one who "smoothed things over" with difficult people. He even recently volunteered to travel to another city to work on a project with a difficult manager. No one else wanted to do it. It made perfect sense to him that he should be the one to go and he was actually looking forward to it. This was a *vasana* (tendency produced by accumulated samskaras) based on an ongoing pattern from his childhood—being the OK one around difficult people. Yet, this thought had never entered his surface mind.

In repeating this pattern, new samskaras from his current difficult relationships are being formed. With John, the new imprints from the activation of the "people around me are not OK" vasana merge with the past imprints and negatively influence his quality of life and his ability to connect with others. Whenever negativity appears in our lives, we must discover the samskara or vasana that is contributing to it so it can change.

It is important to cease identification with the negativity in our minds. In workshops, people often react with surprise when I tell them that negative thoughts and feelings are not really part of us, but the result of the deep mind trying to alert us to a negative samskara that should be removed. Another way of saying this is that negative memories have not been digested and thus have not become dormant. That is why negative memories loom so large and echo in the mind, while positive ones seem to fade. When we fail to see the truth or put things "under the rug," they come back with more force.

The Traya techniques you will learn in chapter 3 pierce the veil between the surface and deep mind by mindfully focusing on a chakra. The deep mind will then alert us to that chakra's undigested samskaras that are producing emotional discomfort or pain. We can then readily surface, digest, and release them.

We can finally leave the past behind and stop reacting to the present as if it were the past. I saw this phenomenon in sessions with Violet, who was complaining about feeling trapped in her marriage. She reported that she had asked her husband for a divorce during an argument. He didn't think that she was serious and told her that she could move on and he wouldn't stop her and would even support her. Now that she was free to do what she wanted, she decided she didn't feel trapped in her marriage anymore so she didn't want to leave. Her feeling of entrapment switched to the town that she lived in (where "nothing was happening") and then to her animals even though she was devoted to them.

"I can't do this or that because of the constraints of living in a 'nothing' town and having pets that force me to be home at a certain time. I feel trapped."

When we explored the "trapped energy" located in the solar plexus chakra, she realized that this was an old feeling generated by her social fears: "My self-consciousness made me feel like a prisoner. I wanted to be so many things but fear held me back."

We continued to explore the memories (samskaras) that created her self-consciousness and fear. She was able to stop looking outside for the sources of her pain—the people, animals, and places in her life, and focus on what was really holding her back—her self-consciousness and fear. Now this material was available to the surface mind and could be digested. Her surface mind was problem solving a need while completely unaware of what was driving the need—"I feel trapped by my fear and I want to free myself." The pain body contained the samskaras causing the fear, the feeling of entrapment, and the false attributions. The deep mind provided the truth: "It is the fear that is trapping me." The following highlights the mind dynamics related to Violet's situation before the healing of the specific samskaras that were contributing to her fear:

Surface Mind

- Negative thoughts and feelings—"I feel trapped."
- Looking for solutions outside

Pain Body

- Samskaras producing trapped feeling and fear
- Samskaras producing false attributions—i.e., blaming marriage, place, animals

Deep Mind

- "Sends up" negative thoughts and feelings to surface mind to draw attention to negative samskaras
- Provides truth to surface mind via Traya—it is fear that is causing sense of entrapment—to begin digestion and healing of fear samskaras

The pain body is not an innate part of our mind. It is an intrusion. Even the most wounded of us can realize that we are created of positive energy, and it is only when one picks up negativity from others or from negative experiences that we feel pain. Every time we heal a samskara, the liberated prana strengthens the positive aspects of the chakras and weakens the pain body. Thus, it can be diminished and even eventually eliminated samskara by samskara. Carl Jung said, "One does not become enlightened by imagining figures of light, but by making the darkness conscious."[3] Traya allows us to go one step further by making the darkness conscious and then *removing* it.

Chapter 3 outlines the Traya mind healing techniques. You can go ahead and read it, of course, but I recommend that you first familiarize yourself with the structure of the subtle body in chapter 2 and then start to work with the chakras by doing the simple mindfulness exercises in that chapter. You can practice the mind stance that is useful when working with the chakras. You will begin to connect to the chakras and learn valuable information about the condition of each. I expect you will also begin to appreciate the deep mind as your ally and teacher as well as the ease of working with it.

••• EXERCISE: OBSERVE THE PAIN BODY •••

Awareness is the first step in healing. Watch your mind and become aware of negative thoughts or feelings the deep mind is sending up. Write down one or two on a page you will save. Observe these thoughts and how you own them or identify with them. Be mindful of the different perspective described above—negative thoughts belong to the "pain body" and our minds are sending them up as flags that something needs to be healed. They are not part of us.

---

3. Carl Gustav Jung, "The Philosophical Tree," *Alchemical Studies, Collected Works*, volume 13, translated by R. F. C. Hull (Princeton, New Jersey: Princeton University Press, 1967), 265.

Chapter 2

THE SUBTLE BODY:
Mindfully Connecting with the Chakras

Mind, body, and spirit are different forms of energy. The mind is energy in wave form and the body is energy in particle form. Think of a radio. The body of the radio is made up of solid particles and the information that plays on the radio arrives in wave form. Spirit is even subtler energy and that is why we are often not aware of it at all, while everyone is aware of mind and body. The subtle or energy body, composed of prana, animates and connects all three of these forms—mind, body, and spirit. It also connects us to other people and all of nature. As you will see, the subtle body is not just a new age interest that is fun to read about—it is the fiber of our being, providing the energy that animates us and the subtle programming that makes us human. Desire, confidence, empathy, ego, intuition, sadness, and fear are just a few of the myriad states of mind formed in the subtle body. If we want to know what makes us think and feel the way we do, we need to become intimate with the subtle body. Then we can cleanse it of unwholesome thoughts, feelings, beliefs, and behaviors.

This chapter provides a basic anatomy of this subtle body and lays the foundation for your Traya work.

More than 2,500 years ago, the ancient Indians, with only their own minds and bodies as research tools, discovered an invisible and subtle body composed of the life energy we call prana existing within the physical body. The Taoists in China also made this discovery perhaps even earlier and called this energy *chi*.

One body is material and easily detectable with the physical senses and the other is composed of prana and invisible. Just as classical physics and quantum physics differ because they each apply to a different form of reality—one macroscopic and one subatomic—the same is true of the gross physical body and the laws that govern its functioning and the finer more subtle laws that govern the subtle body.

Even if the ancients did have MRIs, they wouldn't have been able to see this invisible subtle body and yet they discovered 72,000 *nadis*, subtle channels through which this life energy flows. Later, tantric masters, circa fifth century CE, described subtle energy organs located at major points or plexuses along the spinal axis in the subtle body that both store and move prana. They called them *chakras*, a term that means "wheel" in Sanskrit, as they were thought to spin in a circular motion. Tantric writings reveal a primarily spiritual focus associated with the chakras. Breathing and other techniques designed to stimulate the higher chakras and attain spiritual benefits were used. Knowledge of these chakras and related spiritual practices spread and, over time, various adaptations and modifications appeared. For example, the Vajrayana Buddhist tantra of Tibet was influenced by early tantra.

Primary and Secondary Chakras

There is no authoritative chakra system. Many teachers and sects attribute different qualities and functions to the chakras. They often also differ on how many chakras there are and where they are located in the body. The Indian chakra system includes seven primary chakras aligned along the spine and minor chakras in the limbs and this is the most widespread system. However, my clients have often located issues at points along the spine in addition to the Indian primary chakra locations. As we explored these areas using the techniques described in this book, we found the exact locations of the primary chakras. For example, the heart chakra often depicted between the pectorals over the lower sternum is actually located in the center of the chest. When we found a smaller chakra with a different function than the heart chakra at the sternum, this led to the discovery of an entire secondary chakra subsystem and, after extensive exploration, their functions. Some other systems include chakras other than the seven primary chakras in various locations throughout the body, but none of those systems assign the specific functions to them that we discovered, especially the fact that the functions are related to the nearby primary chakras.

These secondary chakras are located between each of the seven primary chakras and contain aspects related to the neighboring primary chakras located above and below. For example, *manipura*, a primary chakra located at the solar plexus, has the I-consciousness as its function. The heart chakra (*anahata*), located in the center of the chest, has connection to others its function—as we saw in Carolyn's cooking lesson. In between these two chakras at the lower sternum lies *vajrahridaya* (meaning "diamond heart") and has self-esteem as its *only* function. The self-consciousness of the solar plexus chakra is thus bridged with the need for connection at the heart chakra. What creates self-esteem is feeling acknowledged and important to others and thus connected.

The secondary chakras are smaller than the primary chakras and have only one function while the primary chakras have additional attributes. Think of a string of beads strung along our spine from the tops of our heads to the base of our spine. This string has seven large beads interspersed with smaller ones—the large beads are the seven primary chakras and the smaller ones are the seven secondary chakras. Small but potent, the secondary chakras provide a smooth transition between the primary chakra levels of consciousness. For consistency, I have given these secondary chakras Sanskrit names based on their functions in the following list, but throughout this book I refer to them by their function in order to more clearly distinguish them from the primary chakras which are referred to by name or location. Note that between the pelvic chakra (*svadhisthana*) and the solar plexus chakra there lie two secondary chakras instead of just one. Perhaps because this is the farthest distance between any two chakras in the body.

There are also smaller tertiary chakras located off of the spinal axis in the extremities. These serve as conduits of energy in and out of the heart chakra in the center of the chest down the arms and out of the hands and in and out of the root chakra (*muladhara*) to the soles of the feet. Note that all the chakras open in both the front and the back of the body.

Primary (large beads)
7. Crown chakra (sahasrara), top of head, white violet
6. Third eye chakra (ajna), between eyebrow, indigo
5. Throat chakra (vishuddha), center of neck, sky blue
4. Heart chakra (anahata), center of chest, green
3. Solar plexus chakra (manipura), diaphragm, yellow
2. Pelvic chakra (svadhisthana), one inch below navel, orange
1. Root chakra (muladhara), pubic bone, red

Secondary (small beads)
6.5. Insight chakra (satyamanas), center of forehead, violet
5.5. True speech chakra (satyavadya), top of neck, dark blue
4.5. Asking chakra (satyahridaya), top of chest, right below clavicle, blue-green
3.5. Self-esteem chakra (vajrahridaya), sternum, yellow-green
2.75. Release chakra (mukta), halfway between abhaya and manipura, yellow-orange
2.5. Fearless chakra (abhaya), ½ inch above navel, orange-yellow
1.5. Imagination chakra (atiloka), between svadhisthana and muladhara, red-orange

Tertiary
Palms of Hands
Elbow Crook
Back of Knee
Soles of Feet

Primary   Secondary

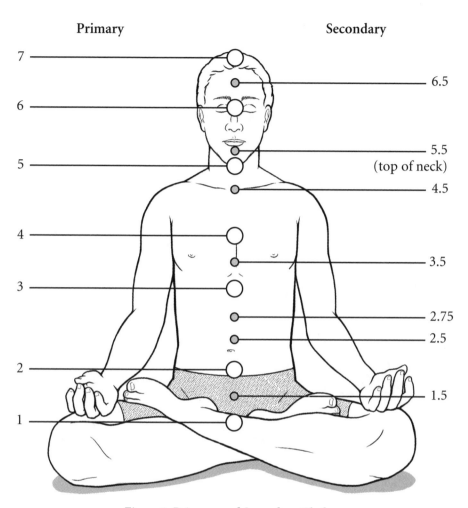

Figure 1: Primary and Secondary Chakras

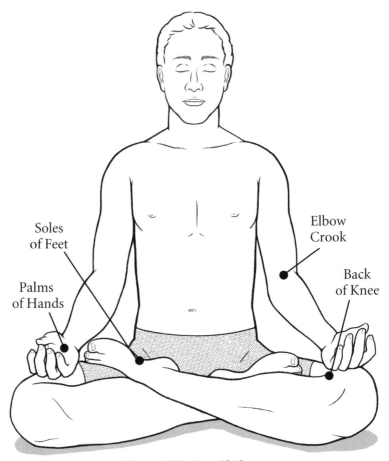

Soles
of Feet

Palms
of Hands

Elbow
Crook

Back
of Knee

Figure 2: Tertiary Chakras

Yukta Triveni (Major Nadis)

There are three central nadis, or channels, that transport prana in the subtle body: *sushumna* is the central nadi that runs along the spine from the base of the spine in the root chakra up to the crown chakra (*sahasrara*) on top of the head. Two other important nadis—*ida* (the sun) and *pingala* (the moon), spiral around sushumna from the root chakra up to the third eye chakra (*ajna*) and between the eyes, where they then reverse direction and proceed out of the nostrils.

Note that the root chakra is the source of the *Yukta Triveni,* or the three central nadis of prana (sushumna, ida, and pingala), in the human body. It is also the dwelling place of *kundalini shakti,* or subtle spiritual energy (also called "spiritual prana"), that when awakened rises up the *sushumna* channel to the crown chakra.

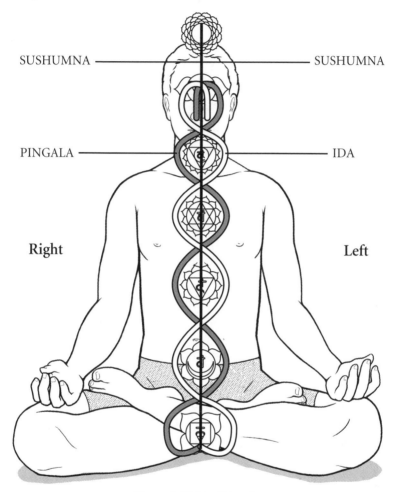

SUSHUMNA ——————————— SUSHUMNA

PINGALA ———————————— IDA

Right   **Left**

Figure 3: Yukta Triveni

Life-Force Energy and the Human Organism

We can see that the subtle body connects into the universal prana through the crown chakra and to earth energy through the root chakra. While all of the chakras take in and give out prana, these are the main places that we "plug in."

Prana animates us. When you go to sleep at night, the body and mind are reinvigorated by the intake of prana in the sleep state. In yoga philosophy, prana has different forms and operates in specific ways in the body/mind:

- **Prana (personal subtype of universal prana):** governs intake, brings in fuel
- **Samana:** governs digestion of food, air, and experiences (whether sensory, emotional, or mental), converts fuel to energy
- **Vyana:** governs circulation of nutrients
- **Apana:** releases waste materials, eliminates toxins
- **Udana:** governs circulation of positive energy created in above process

Our interactions with people and the environment are processed or "digested" in the subtle body by means of the *samana* prana—the prana of digestion. If an experience is positive, it will resonate with the positive nature of the chakras and be fully digested and the associated experience prana will flow freely through the system and become dormant. Experiences contrary to the function of a chakra are not fully digested, and energy toxins form as negative samskaras and remain active. Negative samskaras disrupt the flow of prana and produce tendencies counter to the function of the chakra.

The Traya technique you will learn in chapter 3 increases prana and enhances its flow—both within us and in our interactions with our environment. When the positive aspects of the chakras are active in our lives, not only do we feel better but positive energy plays out in our lives and things always seem to work out.

The Functions and Attributes of the Chakras

The following are lists of the primary, secondary, and tertiary chakras and their functions and attributes. This list defines the Sanskrit name, the chakra location, corresponding natural element, functions, attributes, the pain body impact, the *bija* (seed sound), and color.

Primary Chakras

7TH CHAKRA—SAHASRARA
- **Location:** top of head (crown)
- **English meaning:** thousand-petaled
- **Element:** no earthly element as it is beyond material world
- **Function:** autonomy
- **Attributes:** connection to universe, liberation from false beliefs, freedom, truth filter, vision, elevation, manifestation, wisdom, spiritual maturity, understanding, ebullience, bliss, power, influence
- **Pain body impact:** includes being controlled by outside influences, limited by false beliefs, cannot manifest vision, lacks spiritual understanding
- **Seed sound:** om
- **Color:** violet

6TH CHAKRA—AJNA
- **Location:** between the eyebrows
- **English meaning:** command
- **Element:** no earthly element as it is beyond material world
- **Function:** clear perception
- **Attributes:** clarity, wisdom, intuition, insight, foresight, timing, vision, lucidity, acceptance, truth, wide perspective, resolve, piercing illusions, discernment, detachment, objectivity
- **Pain body impact:** includes denial, lack of perspective, discounting intuition, cannot see or accept truth
- **Seed sound:** hum
- **Color:** indigo

5TH CHAKRA—VISHUDDHA
- **Location:** throat at center of neck
- **English meaning:** pure
- **Element:** ether
- **Function:** self-expression

- **Attributes:** communication, identity, organization, listening, leadership, spontaneity, authenticity, extroversion, wisdom, impact, space, visibility
- **Pain body impact:** difficulty with communication, inauthentic, disorganized, discounts inner voice, follower, lack of spontaneity, poor self-image, hiding
- **Seed sound:** ham
- **Color:** blue

4TH CHAKRA—ANAHATA

- **Location:** center of chest
- **English meaning:** unstruck
- **Element:** air
- **Function:** connection to self, other, nature, and spirit
- **Attributes:** abundance, empathy, enthusiasm, generosity, forgiveness, hope, compassion, fullness, happiness, love, knowledge, motivation, inspiration, confidence, trust, truth, desire, passion, joie de vivre
- **Pain body impact:** feeling empty and disconnected, lack of motivation, fearful, distrustful, sad, uninspired, hopeless, feeling unloved, financial issues
- **Seed sound:** yam
- **Color:** green

3RD CHAKRA—MANIPURA

- **Location:** diaphragm (solar plexus)
- **English meaning:** gem site
- **Element:** fire
- **Function:** I-consciousness
- **Attributes:** ego, intellect, structure, logic, reasoning, will, drive, determination, duality, direction, orientation in time and place, courage, clarity, ease, flexibility, decision-making, problem-solving, calm, engagement, justice, fairness, balance, self-

control, open-mind, vitality, going with the flow, and ability to focus

- **Pain body impact:** too much thinking, fear, worry, sense of isolation, disengaged, distracted, willful, controlling, critical, judgmental, confused, difficulty with decisions, inflated ego, black and white and/or extreme thinking, compulsive, reactive, disorientation, dependence on intellect, distant, irritable, impatient, inflexible, guilt
- **Seed sound:** ram
- **Color:** yellow

2ND CHAKRA—SVADHISTHANA

- **Location:** pelvis, one inch below navel
- **English meaning:** own abode
- **Element:** water
- **Function:** personal power in relationships
- **Attributes:** boundaries, emotions, creativity, sexual energy, centeredness, poise, charisma, buoyancy, humor, dignity
- **Pain body impact:** codependence, suppressed anger, suppressed or misdirected sexual energy, lack of creative energy, poor boundaries, passive, not centered, boredom
- **Seed sound:** vam
- **Color:** orange

1ST CHAKRA—MULADHARA

- **Location:** base of spine
- **English meaning:** root support
- **Element:** earth
- **Function:** embodiment
- **Attributes:** grounding, safety, security, doing, action, movement, standing up for self, accomplishment, moment connection, kundalini, manifestation

- **Pain body impact:** disembodiment, feeling unsafe, difficulty doing and accomplishing, dependent, lack of attention to detail, spacey, ungrounded, difficulty overcoming obstacles or moving forward
- **Seed sound:** lam
- **Color:** red

Secondary Chakras

CHAKRA 6.5—SATYAMANAS

Location: between ajna and sahasrara

English meaning: turn the mind toward the truth

Function: insight into truth

Color: violet

CHAKRA 5.5—SATYAVADYA

Location: between vishuddha and ajna

English meaning: speak the truth

Function: true speech

Color: dark blue

CHAKRA 4.5—SATYAHRIDAYA

Location: between anahata and vishuddha

English meaning: heart truth

Function: express or ask for what the heart wants

Color: blue-green

CHAKRA 3.5 VAJRAHRIDAYA

Location: between manipura and anahata

English meaning: diamond heart

Function: self-esteem

Color: yellow-green

CHAKRA 2.75 MUKTA

Location: between abhaya and manipura

English meaning: to let go

Function: full letting go or release of physical tension and false defenses based on fear

Color: yellow-orange

CHAKRA 2.5 ABHAYA

Location: between svadhisthana and mukta

English meaning: without fear

Function: unafraid of others' power

Color: orange-yellow

CHAKRA 1.5 ATILOKA

Location: between muladhara and svadhisthana

English meaning: to rise above the material world

Function: lifts psyche beyond the mundane to magical aspects of life provided by people

Color: red-orange

Tertiary Chakras

- **Soles of feet:** connects muladhara to earth energy (grounding)
- **Behind knees:** helps move energy from muladhara to soles of feet
- **Palms of hands:** connects anahata (healing) energy to places on one's own or others' bodies through the palms of the hands
- **Elbow crook:** assists in channeling anahata energy to palms and outward from there

Mindfully Connecting with the Chakras

Traya is a mindfulness practice in which we become mindful of the subtle body and its contents and functions. We realize that we have already experienced sensations produced by samskaras in the chakras, but we may not have specifically recognized them as such. There are three locations in particular: the throat chakra where we may at times feel a sensation of tightness or a lump; the heart chakra where we can feel a squeezing or heaviness in the chest in certain circumstances; and the solar plexus where we can at times feel a clenching or knot in the stomach area. These are all signs that there are negative samskaras in those areas. Our goal is to approach the subtle body directly and become mindful of it in a different way.

At first you may need a tool to help you turn inward and cross the chasm created by our cultural tendency of being externally focused. The following two exercises act as bridges that will facilitate your passage. Once you arrive at your destination for the first time, you may be met tentatively. Don't worry. Like an explorer approaching a village for the first time, you may find that the inhabitants hang back, but when you return they will come out to meet you. In future journeys you won't need to travel far, as the subtle body will meet you on the road bearing gifts. Even paying the slightest attention to the subtle body is a giant step in the process of awakening and healing.

••• EXERCISE: SOUND BRIDGE •••
TO THE CHAKRAS

One of the best ways to sense the vibrations and stimulate the chakras is with sound. Tantric masters associated certain bijas, or seed sounds, with each chakra. When chanted either aloud or silently, they activate the related chakra and allow us to connect with them.

Starting with the root chakra at the base of the spine, focus your attention at that location and chant its seed sound, LAM, over and over. Very slowly draw out the sound. Next do this with the pelvic chakra about one inch below the navel and chant VAM. Continue to the solar plexus chakra at the diaphragm RAM and to the remaining chakras: heart, YAM; throat, HAM; third eye, HUM; and crown, OM.

It is quite impressive how these sounds actually do connect to their related chakras. Test it out. Pick any one at random and repeat that sound either aloud or silently and notice how its related chakra is stimulated in the subtle body and how your mind is drawn to that location.

••• EXERCISE: SCENES FROM NATURE •••
(LANDSCAPES OF THE MIND)

If you were impressed by the relationship of certain sounds to particular chakras, you will be amazed by the mind's connection to nature and its use of nature images to convey information to us. Connecting with a chakra and obtaining information in the Traya process requires a mindful stance. This exercise will help you to become comfortable with that stance before attempting to identify samskaras in the Traya practice later on. You will learn more about that in chapter 3. The basics here are very useful for obtaining information regarding the health of a chakra.

The solar plexus chakra provides a tendency to separate, take apart, and see things as separate from us. We see ourselves as separate not only from each other but from nature also. We know from science that the physical material of our bodies comes directly from the elements released at the beginning of our universe. Now we will see that our minds also have a deep connection to nature and the basic elements— earth, water, fire, air, and ether.

Tantric philosophy teaches that the human microcosm is a reflection of the universal macrocosm, and in this exercise we see the truth of that viewpoint. The Traya healing process is about reconnecting with our body, mind, and spirit and understanding how we are part of rather than separate from. We see there is really no separation between inside and outside.

Our connection to nature becomes readily apparent when we understand the physical elements and their relationship to our psyche. For example, one can see with the "inner eye" a particular scene from nature at each of the first five chakras that have a material element associated with them. The two higher chakras, third eye and crown, are energetically beyond the material earthly realm and are connected more to the universal energies and, therefore, have no earthbound landscapes associated with them. Some associate even subtler ethereal energy with each.

The presence or absence in the scene that appears of the element associated with one of the "lower" five chakras will give valuable and dependable information regarding the amount of samskaric material present. I have found that these scenes are representative for everyone and are good tools for approximating the type of dominant energy in any of the chakras and, therefore, the general state of mind of the person.

The following list shows the seven primary chakras, their associated elements and the scenes associated with positive and negative mind states.

Crown (Sahasrara)

- Element: no associated earthly elements
- Scenes for positive mind states: no associated scenes from nature
- Scenes for negative mind states: no associated scenes from nature

Third Eye (Ajna)

- Element: no associated earthly elements
- Scenes for positive mind states: no associated scenes from nature
- Scenes for negative mind states: no associated scenes from nature

Throat (Vishuddha)

- Element: ether
- Scenes for positive mind states: wide open blue sky
- Scenes for negative mind states: enclosed space with no sky

Heart (Anahata)

- Element: air
- Scenes for positive mind states: open landscapes with lots of green grass and bright sun
- Scenes for negative mind states: darkness and/or water

Solar Plexus (Manipura)

- Element: fire
- Scenes for positive mind states: open space with bright yellow sun, desert
- Scenes for negative mind states: darkness and/or water

Pelvis (Svadhisthana)

- Element: water
- Scenes for positive mind states: rapidly flowing body of water
- Scenes for negative mind states: dry, cracked earth, desert

Root (Muladhara)

- Element: earth
- Scenes for positive mind states: solid earth
- Scenes for negative mind states: water or mud

Note that the list above shows the extremes of the range. For example, the wide open cloudless blue sky for the throat chakra represents ether or sky energy without obstructions. All the positive attributes of this chakra will be apparent in the person's life who has this scene at the throat. They will have excellent communication energy and a strong sense of identity.

Alternatively, the enclosed space without sky represents the opposite extreme and the negative aspects of an intensely samskaric throat chakra will be apparent in that person's life—perhaps significant difficulty being heard or seen. Variations representing some, but not total, obstruction will present as a mixed bag—maybe a cloudy sky, or high mountains with little sky, etc.

The key in the visualized scene is to discern the presence or absence of the element. Again, this reflects the state of that chakra and the presence or absence of a chakra's positive or negative attributes. For example, if one sees a snowy or icy scene in the heart, we know that there is loneliness there and one feels "left out in the cold" or disconnected. Or if one sees a flower at the solar plexus, there is neither water nor sun but we know that a flower requires sun so there is a hint that suggests the chakra is samskaric but not extremely so—i.e., there is no water visible.

Note that while I use the scenes as additional information when working with self or others, sometimes the progression of the changes is not as clear as we would like it in the scenes. Use it as a general guide not an absolute one as before the chakra is purified, a scene may revert to a negative temporarily. The primary determinant of the status of a chakra is always how one thinks and feels and what is going on in one's life.

I also like to use the nature scenes with clients so that I can better judge their state of mind and so they can have the experience of working with and trusting the deep mind. Very anxious people can sometimes present looking calm and collected, for example, yet the scene they report at the solar plexus chakra is a water scene which gives me a better idea of their actual state of mind as the water indicates the opposite—a significantly fearful mind.

When working with the Traya process healing the negative aspects of a chakra, the scene will steadily improve as the mind improves. Suppose, for example, the first scene at the solar plexus chakra is a waterfall and you work with it and then the scene will change over time to a lake (still water but calmer), then a puddle, and then eventually dry land and sunshine, reflecting the solar plexus chakra's healthy fire energy. However, when going from a significantly negative to a positive scene, it takes time for the positive scene to stabilize. A significantly negative scene reveals that there are many samskaras in the chakra. You may release some samskaras and get a positive scene but then the energy settles and a negative one may reappear. Keep going until the positive scene sticks. Of course, you will notice the positive impact on your mind also and that is always the final determinant.

Remember that none of us knows what it is like to be *completely* free of samskaras. For example, if we are not grounded in our bodies, we don't know what that is like and we may be satisfied when we feel more grounded without having attained complete grounding. Thus, we may be unaware that there is still room for improvement in a chakra that is more positive than negative but not completely healthy. That is where the scenes are most helpful. Don't quit working with a chakra until you see a positive scene over a period of time. They are a road map to becoming completely human and reaching our full potential.

Chakra Diagnostics

Sit in any comfortable seated posture with the spine erect—on a chair is fine. Close your eyes and focus your attention on the soles of your feet. Imagine that you can breathe in and out through the minor chakras on the soles of your feet for a minute or two. This grounds our consciousness in the body and in the moment.

1. Become mindful of a chakra by focusing your attention on the location of a chakra in your body. Let's use your solar plexus chakra located at your diaphragm to start.

2. Imagine that there is an opening there that you can breathe in and out of. Focus your attention there and start breathing in and out as if the breath were actually going in and out of the opening. Soft, gentle breath.

Think of what it is like to tune to a radio station. When you tune the dial to a certain station, the scheduled radio program plays. When you "tune in" to a particular chakra by focusing your attention on it, it too will "play" by responding to requests for information.

While focusing on the chakra, let a scene from nature appear in your mind. Note that this is not a visualization exercise. The mind doesn't need your help but rather it needs for you to get out of the way. So your only job is to keep your attention focused on the "opening" in the chakra, gently breathe in and out, and be mindful of any scene that appears in your mind without searching, choosing, or editing. Note the scene and open your eyes. The solar plexus chakra is fire energy so any amount of water or darkness here will signify the presence of some negative aspects, such as worry or fear and/or too much thinking. Additionally, with all the chakras, a wide open space is always important.

People often say, "But if I know what scene is supposed to be there, won't this interfere with the information that comes?" No. The information is coming from the deep mind and you cannot control the deep mind. It operates according to truth and, as long as you open to it mindfully and stay out of the way, it will communicate the truthful scene.

Try this exercise and then cross-reference the scene information you obtain with the lists showing the positive and negative attributes of a chakra and see if it reflects how you are actually thinking and feeling.

I suggest that you work with these sound and scene exercises for a bit before moving on to the next chapter. It is not an absolute requirement but will help you to connect with the chakras with the appropriate mind stance—getting out of your own way and "letting" the information surface. You may also come to experience the deep mind as ally and teacher that is providing you with crucial information. You will also appreciate the ease of working with it before we explore the chakras in more depth with the Traya techniques.

Chapter 3

THE BASIC TRAYA TECHNIQUE
AND WAYS TO USE IT

In this chapter, I describe the Traya process that allows for direct engagement with the subtle body and its healing mechanisms. We saw
in chapter 1 that each chakra manages a part of the mind and negative experiences that aren't resonant with the function of a chakra will
produce a samskara, or negative energy imprint, in the chakra. These
samskaras remain undigested and distort the functions of the chakras.
As a result, they end up producing negative thoughts, behaviors, and
feelings—the pain body. To turn on the mind's innate healing mechanism, we need to reconnect with the samskaric energy in the subtle
body, digest it, and release it.

In the mind, digestion equals recognizing and acknowledging
the truth. We also saw that many truths of experience lie in the deep
mind, out of reach of the surface mind, and just recalling on an intellectual or even emotional level is not enough. In the Traya process,
the veil between the surface mind and the deep mind is lifted and a
whole new world of information opens up to us. The barrier between
what is in the mind versus what is on the mind is pierced. Traya allows the deep mind to be heard and it has a lot to say.

We begin to understand puzzling feelings and behaviors—why we
feel afraid when the boss comes into the room even though he or she
is really nice and supportive, or why we are so impatient with our
children even though we promise ourselves we won't be. The chakras

become accessible and understandable as they teach us. We can even put aside whatever information about the chakras we have been exposed to, as we don't need to know anything about a chakra in order to work with it. In fact, we may get in our own way if we have too many preconceived ideas.

Let me emphasize that this is a user-friendly process. As we connect with the chakras, we connect with our innate wisdom that is always guiding us toward wholeness. We soon see that Traya is an organic process supported and encouraged by the higher intelligence within all of us. Interaction with the chakras is not only practical and productive but also uplifting and inspiring.

At first the chakra functions and how the memories connect to a chakra may not be so clear. As you work with them, their impact and the subtleties of the chakra functions and attributes become clearer. Like meditation, you can't understand it intellectually. You can only understand it by experiencing it over time, discovering new dimensions and truths as you go. Optimally, you have a regular meditation practice and have experienced observing thoughts without attaching to them. If not, you can start where you are. Many people I have worked with have no experience with meditation at all but readily take to this process.

The following is an overview of the Traya techniques, including variations on the basic method. Read the information over first. In part 2, the exercises related to each chakra will help you put these techniques into practice.

The Basic Traya Technique

Following is the Traya technique for removing negative samskaras from the mind. This is where we get the basics of the practice in five simple steps:

- **Step 1: Mindfulness and Focus**—Tune in to a chakra.
- **Step 2: Surface**—See what memories it brings to the surface of your mind.

- **Step 3: Release**—Visualize the negative energy moving out of your chakra.
- **Step 4: Replace and Imprint**—Visualize positive energy replacing the negative energy that has been released and receive the positive imprint.
- **Step 5: Diagnostic Scene from Nature**—Let your chakra reveal a scene from nature. You can diagnose its message using the elements and the scenes associated with the chakra and its positive and negative mind states. This step is optional.

Please ground yourself at the start and again at the finish of the Traya practice by focusing on the soles of the feet and breathing in and out of an imaginary opening there.

As with meditation, we don't have to be perfect; we just do the best we can. Remember, the mind wants to heal and when you go toward it, it will come toward you. As I always say to my students, don't worry, there is no right and wrong and if it doesn't work at first, there are ways to get it going. The most important advice I have is to keep it simple and get out of your own way. It is like a free association through the body. Getting out of your own way means not actively looking for anything or rejecting anything that comes. Just observe. If you skipped them, I'd suggest going back to the sound and scene exercises in the preceding chapter so you will have some experience with the mindful, non-interfering approach helpful for this work. It is good to ground oneself in the body at the beginning and end of each Traya session. Do this by sitting up straight, focusing on the soles of your feet, and breathing in and out gently with your attention there.

Step 1: Mindfulness and Focus

Sit in any comfortable seated posture with your spine erect and your feet flat on the floor if sitting in a chair. Close your eyes and focus attention on the soles of your feet. Imagine that you can breathe in and out through the minor chakras in the soles of your feet for a minute or two. This will ground your consciousness in the body and in the moment.

Next, focus your attention on the location of a chakra in your body. Let's use the solar plexus chakra located at the diaphragm to start.

Imagine that there is an opening there that you can breathe in and out of. Concentrate your attention there and start breathing in and out as if the breath were actually going in and out of the opening. Soft, gentle breath.

Step 2: Surface

Returning to the radio analogy, when you "tune in" to a particular chakra, it too will "play" by sending memories up to the surface mind. The impetus is always toward healing, so the mind will "send up" an experience that has produced a negative samskara. Please don't search for anything. You don't have to do anything to get the radio program to play. Just listen. Let it come up like a bubble coming up through the water. I repeat because it is important—the mind doesn't need your help but rather it needs for you to get out of the way. Your only job is to keep your attention focused on the "opening" in the chakra, gently breathe in and out, and be mindful of any memories or other material that come into your awareness.

Ask, "What memories are here that are ready to come to the surface?"

Sometimes the memory comes fully formed and sometimes a piecemeal "hook" will appear. For example, you may remember a particular object, person, or place. Stay with that and ask for more information until the complete memory unfolds. Don't reject anything as unimportant or unrelated but stay open and mindful, and you will learn as you go. Even a seemingly unimportant image or issue is there for a reason. Big or small doesn't matter. For example, Paul recently remembered a checkered tablecloth, then when staying with it, remembered a craft sale he and a few friends had in second grade near a store in the mall. The tablecloth was covering the card table. Still the full memory didn't come. He stayed with it and then remembered that an adult bluntly told him that his piece was overpriced. He felt humiliated in front of his friends. This came up in the solar plexus chakra because he felt the judgment of others.

Raina felt a sense of sadness instead of a memory. When she focused on the heart chakra, she didn't get a memory at first but rather she described, "Sad feeling—a cap on something that doesn't want to come off—gorilla. A nebulous feeling of being incapable of getting excited."

Since we know that every negative thought or feeling results from experience precursors, I asked, "What memories are here that contributed to this?" Then the deep mind with the associated samskara responded:

> …I was squashed a lot when excited—I was told, "You can't have it or do that."

If working with a chakra and a memory doesn't come immediately, be patient and inquisitive and the information will come. After you learn the basic Traya process, you can review the additional methods later in this chapter. Note that Traya will surface memories regardless of when they happened if they are significant for healing. If they are from very early childhood and the memory comes piecemeal, you may have to stay with it until it unfolds completely. Since everything registers in the deep mind, even these early childhood experiences will come with relevant associations.

Step 3: Release

The next step is to visualize the "negative energy" related to the samskara going out of the opening of the chakra; the apana prana that eliminates toxins from the system will remove it. Remember: Your mind put it there and your mind can take it away.

Note that with this "release" step and the next "replace" step a more active visualization process is called for. There is still some "letting," as with letting a memory surface on its own, but when I say "visualize," this calls for a slightly more active process and it is OK to be less passive and more engaged with these steps. For this solar plexus chakra, some people visualize liquids or sludge and some visualize solids like rocks. Whatever feels right for you is fine. The memory will remain but without the negative energetic charge, and it can now proceed to a dormant state of storage. If there is resistance and the negative energy doesn't seem to "want" to flow out, ask for more information—"What else do I need to know?" This will often get things moving.

As we gain experience removing individual memory samskaras, we will become even more aware of how they contributed to our painful thoughts, feelings, and behaviors.

Samskaras may surface one at a time in the beginning and then after we gain experience they will sometimes come as a string of memories. It is not necessary to wait until the outflow stops before surfacing the next one. It is best to get the flow going with the first memory, and as that goes out, let the next memory appear in your mind and add that negative energy to the flow. After you finish surfacing memories, you can expel all of the remaining energy by visualizing it all going out and just wait for it to stop—usually a minute or two.

Step 4: Replace and Imprint

The sun and sunshine have been recognized by the ancients in India as sources of positive prana, and we are going to use the image of sunlight filled with prana to replace the samskaras that have been expelled from the chakra.

Briefly visualize positive energy in the form of light coming directly from the sun and flowing into the chakra, filling the space left by the negative samskaric energy that dissipated.

Next, as this positive prana flows in, take the passive, letting stance and ask, "What is this positive energy bringing into my life?" Note the words that appear in your mind as the higher intelligence provides some positive reinforcement via the Inner Ear, the part of the mind that hears the words of the higher intelligence or Inner Teacher. These words make a positive imprint on the mind and emphasize the point that the negativity has just changed to something positive. Once you get a word or two, move to step 5 or ground yourself by breathing in and out through the tertiary chakras in the soles of your feet.

Step 5: Diagnostic Scene from Nature (Optional)
While keeping focus on the chakra, gently breathe in and out, let a scene from nature appear in your mind, and note the presence or absence of the chakra element. This helps to actually "see" changes appearing in the chakra. As we learned in chapter 2, as we remove samskaras the associated chakra element will become more dominant. Again, these are: throat chakra, ether; heart chakra, air; solar plexus chakra, fire; pelvic chakra, water; root chakra, earth.

An Example of the Basic Traya Technique

Step 1: Mindfulness and Focus

- Choose a chakra. In this example we will focus on the solar plexus chakra.
- Focus attention there and take a passive, letting stance.

Step 2: Surface

- Ask for memories. What memories are here?
- Take a passive, letting stance.
- Note the memory—e.g., "I was often criticized at the family dinner table."

Step 3: Release

- Release negative energy. Visualize energy going out in any form. Common ones are sludge, rocks, etc.
- You can be more active with visualization here.

Step 4: Replace and Imprint

- Replace the negative with positive energy and positive imprint. Visualize positive energy in the form of light coming in and taking up space vacated by the negative that went out.
- Ask, "What is this positive energy bringing in with it?"
- Note any words that you receive: calm, ease, etc.

- You can be more active with visualizing the light.
- Take a passive, letting stance.

Step 5: Scene from Nature (Optional)

- Note the optimal scene from nature—e.g., solar plexus chakra shows a hot, sunny scene.
- Visualize a scene from nature for this chakra.
- Note presence or absence of chakra element. (Covered in chapter 2.)
- Take a passive, letting stance.

Note that in the above only one memory is surfaced for illustrative purposes. In practice, both steps 2 and 3 are repeated until you feel that enough memories are surfaced for this session, and then after you feel that the negative outflow has stopped, you move on to steps 4 and 5. You can then end the Traya practice by bringing your attention back to the soles of your feet and breathing in and out a few times to help ground yourself.

Please note that this is *not* a process based on emotional catharsis. Sometimes emotions will appear but often not. Since we are approaching experiences through the subtle body and not the emotional body, reliving the emotions of the negative situation is *not* necessary for healing. If you are dealing with a significant pain body and there is some emotional disassociation, reintegration happens in sync with the later stages of growth. Of course, when you work with sensitive energy, such as heart chakra energy, you may feel some of the associated emotions, but because of the approach through the subtle body, strong emotions are often mitigated. If a strong emotion comes up, pay attention to it, feel it in your body, and acknowledge it, and it will soon pass.

It is enough to surface and release the samskaric memory energy from the subtle body. With the memory comes truth and insight—this is the impact on me. This is enough for the samana prana digestion process to work. It is always the truth that heals. Udana prana then releases the new positive energy into the subtle energy system.

Note that a chakra can be out of balance in two ways. It can be overactive or underactive. The pelvic chakra, for example, has the attribute of humor energy. Relating to others through constant joking would be an example of an overactive attribute. Being dour and humorless, on the other hand, reveals an underactive attribute.

The above is the basic version of the chakra exploration that I have used over the years. If you are persistent, and it will take time, you will be bountifully rewarded. Negativity will leave your mind and peace and joy will appear along with the other positive aspects of the chakras. You will see the depths of your conditioning and have some compassion for yourself and others. In the future if you get caught up in any habitual pattern, you will not only see it from a new perspective but you will be happy to see it because you know now that you can change it.

More Ways to Use Traya to Target Samskaras

In the basic approach given previously, samskaras were identified by focusing on a chakra and asking, "What memories are here?" You can also locate samskaras by tracing them back to their origins in various ways, which I'll outline here. These are all simply different ways to locate samskaras in the subtle body and would be done prior to or as part of step 1 of the basic Traya technique. Once the location of the samskara is identified, step 1 would proceed and then, the rest of the Traya steps would then follow.

Manifestation Technique

Remember that the subtle body operates according to the inside/outside rule—what is inside is manifested outside. So if there are negative samskaras in a chakra, then we will see the manifestation of that negativity in our minds and in our lives.

Suppose you are aware of an abiding sense of isolation or disengagement—a manifestation you notice within yourself. You also notice that the people in your life tend to be self-involved and busy—a manifestation in your life. There are different ways to follow this up and ascertain the source so you can heal this dynamic. For example, you could check the primary chakras list in chapter 2 where we out-lined the functions of each of the seven main chakras. Then connect that sense of isolation to a particular chakra—in this case the solar plexus chakra. Focus your attention at the solar plexus (diaphragm) and ask, "What samskaras are here that are contributing to this sense of isolation?"

You can also do this by noticing the lack of something in your mind. Joy, for example; you realize that you don't have very much "joy energy," so you look at the chart and see which chakra produces joy and focus there—the heart chakra in this case.

Following the Body

Instead of looking at the chart, we can let our deep mind or Inner Teacher lead the way. With the first two approaches—the basic and manifestation—we consciously chose where to work by focusing on a particular chakra at random or by relating to something on the chart that needs work and then working on that chakra. We can also let the deep mind signal us through the body. Actually, it may already be sig-naling you. If you feel a "lump" in your throat, a clenching at the solar plexus, or a tightness in the chest, your deep mind is trying to signal that work needs to be done there.

Or you can think about an issue (in this case the isolation). While sitting quietly with your eyes closed, focus on your body, and ask, "Where in me is the energy related to this?" You will feel a sensation of pressure, contraction, or heaviness at one of the chakras or you will be drawn to a specific location. If it is in more than one place, as it often is, select one of them to work with and then go back later and complete the Traya process again at the other location or locations.

With this approach there is the added benefit of experiencing the deep mind as a healing force directing us to material that needs to be expunged. The mind will always respond, and after a while, you will sense a new ally—your Inner Teacher—assisting you with this process. After you have been working with Traya for a period, you may notice that this information may come to you unbidden while you are meditating. In meditation you are connecting to the subtle body and it may alert you to somewhere that needs work—a heaviness at the chest or tightening in the throat for example. This can be addressed after the meditation with Traya.

Following Memories

You can also do Traya with negative memories you are aware of. Suppose you are aware of feeling like an outsider in school when you were young. Follow it back to one of the chakras by becoming mindful of the body and noting any sensations of pressure, contraction, or heaviness as you ask, "Where in me is there any energy related to this issue?" Again, if you are drawn to more than one chakra, choose one. You can always work with the others another time. You can also follow memories by associating them with a particular chakra and working there.

As you read part 2 of this book, you will become familiar with both the attributes of each chakra and the types of experiences that create samskaras in each. When you get to that discussion, if you recognize that you have had a similar type of experience, you can work to release it from the related chakra.

Dreams

I always honor dreams as they are direct communications from the deep mind urging us to address and release specific material. All dreams are significant, but if you have a nightmare or a dream that wakes you up in the middle of the night or otherwise makes you uncomfortable, that is a sign of the deep mind's urgency in removing this material. Don't worry about the content of the dream (no you don't really want to kill your best friend) as the psyche often exaggerates in order to get your attention, make a point as to how important something is, and ensure that you will remember it for follow-up. With dreams, focus on the body and ask, "Where in me are there memories that this dream wants to surface?" Again, you will feel a sensation at one or more of the chakras, focus there and then continue with the basic Traya technique. The more that you respect and work with this valuable information provided by the psyche, the more it will work with you; so keep a pen and pencil next to your bed.

Past-Life Memories

A memory from a previous life will usually only arise if there was a premature (and often violent) death associated with it. Wait until you have experience with the basic Traya until you pursue these memories. If one does come up unbidden, just stay with it until the full circumstances are revealed. Sometimes you need to ask, "And then what happened?" in order to get the full picture.

The Pathwork Technique—Working with Goals

I often use the pathwork tool, which allows one to progress in reaching a specific goal. It is somewhat similar to a visualization exercise, but it is not visualization. With visualization one imagines. With the pathwork one *allows* an image to appear. Similar to the diagnostic scenes from nature we learned about in chapter 2, they arise from within, without any interference from us. This image enables you to see how you are progressing. Does the road that you see allow for rapid *movement* such as an unimpeded highway? Are you on this road? Are you standing, walking, or driving? These indicate how much energy is on the path or if something is preventing you from moving forward or slowing you down. If you are not racing forward on a flat road or even flying a plane (lots of movement), then some of the energy is tied up in samskaras in the chakras and the pathwork helps to identify and release them allowing you to move forward toward your goal.

The key to the pathwork is that the mind uses movement to convey the crucial information. The path image will change as energy is freed up.

••• EXERCISE: •••
THE PATHWORK TECHNIQUE

Sit in the Traya position (spine erect, feet flat on the floor).

Step 1: Image. Breathe in and out gently and allow the image of a path leading to a particular goal, such as finding the right career, to appear in your mind. Try to accept whatever appears, even if it is not your idea of a proper path.

Step 2: Focus. Bring the attention to the body and ask, "Where in me is the energy that is slowing this path down?" One or more chakras will respond with a sensation, signaling that the offending samskaras are in that chakra(s). Once located, the remaining Traya steps are followed—surface, release, and replace.

Resistance

If you are having difficulty getting memories, use the "Following Memories" technique described on page 49. You can bring to mind a negative memory that you can associate with a particular chakra. For example, you grew up in an unsafe and dangerous area of the city and you remember how scary it was to walk to school. This memory can be associated with and released from the root chakra (safety and security in the environment). As you surface and release that memory, stay with it and others will follow. After you finish the complete Traya process, you will notice a deeper connection to your body and the moment—the positive attributes of this chakra. Working with conscious memories often "loosens things up" and starts the process working when it is not flowing naturally.

As noted in chapter 1, most samskaras consist of experiences we are aware of. It is the impact and nuances of these experiences that tend to elude us. From time to time something we had never noticed may come to consciousness.

Repetitive Memories

Sometimes one may become frustrated if the same memory or similar types of memories keep coming up. This will happen if the memory carries a strong charge or is representative of a string of similar memories (e.g., bullied throughout school has an impact in different chakras). Remember that we do not always know all the nuances of the effects and it may have to be surfaced several times to heal all of them. Every time it comes up and energy is released, it is weakened and will eventually stop surfacing. You can always ask, "Why does this keep coming up?" and see how the Inner Teacher responds. All the answers are inside of you. Always remember that the purpose of this process is to move the energy, heal the chakra, and diminish the pain body. If a memory keeps coming up there, is a reason for it.

Traya in Therapy

If you feel you need even more assistance as you move through certain issues, Traya is also applicable in a more traditional type of psychotherapy. The therapeutic relationship is healing in itself. If your therapist is open to it, using this book as a guide, you can do some Traya in your sessions or on your own between sessions. Besides the main benefit of healing negativity in the mind, there are many other benefits to using Traya in therapy and/or between sessions:

1. As we saw in chapter 1, the surface mind does not have direct access to deep mind material. Feelings are more in sync with the deep mind but one is not always in touch with what a feeling is pointing to. Traya allows for direct access to relevant deep mind material and will move a therapy along nicely.

2. Traya provides a cause and effect relationship between memories and current situations that may not otherwise be so clear. It also allows for access to memories long forgotten or discounted.

3. Traya highlights material that may otherwise be overlooked or minimized, such as important nuances of past experiences or early childhood material.

4. Traya reveals underlying truths and encourages self-trust.

5. Traya moves the therapy along by resolving issues and moving the focus to new ones.

6. Traya incorporates the mind-body-spirit connection, extending the reach of the therapy.

Traya in therapy sessions lasts 45–50 minutes, as with a normal session. The usual format is the first 15–20 minutes are discussion, the second 20 minutes are devoted to Traya practice, and the final 10 are wrap-ups.

The Inner Teacher

While Traya is predominantly a healing practice, it is also a spiritual one, because it deepens our connection to the self and our Inner Teacher. The Inner Teacher is the messenger of the higher mind that moves us to heal and grow spiritually. The beauty of Traya is that the Inner Teacher is readily accessible and actively involved in Traya practice and provides an antidote to the negative voice of the pain body. We just need to step out of the surface mind and there it is. The Inner Teacher communicates with us in various ways during Traya practice. It might do so through the body by physical sensations pointing to areas we need to work on, like when we ask, "Where in me is the negative energy?" and we feel a strong sensation at a particular chakra. Or the Inner Teacher might communicate through encouraging positive imprints, diagnostic scenes that provide valuable information on the state of the chakra, or with relevant memories. Some other ways include providing information and guidance in Pathwork, guidance when we ask questions of the Inner Teacher directly, or when information comes through intuition, or even through revealing spiritual truths as we proceed in our Traya practice.

The Inner Teacher is aligned with truth and it is important to respect and value the information it provides. Sometimes it speaks in words and sometimes in images providing support, encouragement, information, and direction. As you proceed with Traya, and you also meditate further, opening the channels of communication with the Inner Teacher, you will come to trust and depend on the wisdom and guidance you receive. This is the most important relationship you will ever have.

Traya is a system of self-investigation that leads to transformation, mastery, and realization. It is a personal practice of lifting negativity from our mind. Several approaches have been discussed above. If I notice that I have a tendency to put others' needs before my own or worry too much about what others think, I would want to find out where this comes from and change it. I would work on the pelvic chakra until I notice that I no longer think or behave like that. If I want to strengthen my singing voice or my ability to speak up in groups, I would work on the throat chakra. If I feel my will, drive, or determination is weak because I tend to lose interest in projects—the solar plexus chakra. If I notice that I have a tendency to fib, spin a story a little too much, or am reluctant to speak the truth when involved in a disagreement, I would work with the true speech chakra (*satyavadya*). If you are feeling stuck in an area of your life, you can use the Pathwork goal-oriented technique. Some of the techniques rely on information provided by the Inner Teacher when we ask, "Where in me is the memory that needs to surface?" and a sensation leads us to a particular location.

Regardless of the best circumstances, no one escapes the formation of negative samskaras. With Traya you can directly address your shortcomings or discomforts so you can live a richer life free of negative thoughts, feelings, and beliefs.

Set some time aside to work with samskaras, preferably daily, but at least several times a week, for fifteen or more minutes using any of the Traya techniques. The exercises in part 2 will help guide you in the beginning. Hopefully, the practice will become as important and integrated into your life as brushing your teeth. Even if you only remove one or two samskaras each session, you will soon notice a positive change. You now have the power and ability to heal your mind and improve and elevate your life in the process.

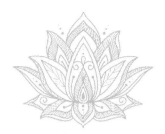

Chapter 4

SUPPORT FOR YOUR TRAYA PRACTICE:
Meditation and Yoga

Now that you have an understanding of how the mind connects with the energy body and how we can make therapeutic use of that with the Traya process, we will move on to a discussion of two practices that can support your work: meditation and yoga. Traya will also support your yoga and meditation practice in many ways but, primarily, by helping you to become more engaged, active, and embodied. All three practices direct us inward, engage the subtle body, and calm, center, and balance the mind. While each are complete practices in themselves, when done in tandem there is increased benefit to each. It is my experience to incorporate all three, but like yoga and meditation, Traya can be a stand-alone practice.

Meditation

If you have a regular meditation practice, you are used to taking time out for spiritual practice, and adding on ten or fifteen minutes of Traya will probably not be a big deal. In addition, meditation prepares the mind for Traya work nicely in that it makes the individual inwardly focused and stimulates the subtle body energy.

Padmasana (lotus pose), the traditional cross-legged meditation posture, is a *mudra*. A mudra is a specific gesture or pose that affects the flow of prana in the body. Here is how padmasana, or any cross-legged seated meditation pose affects the pranic flow: the crossed legs and opened hips activate the root chakra where the Yukta Triveni, or three streams of prana, originate—the sushumna nadi, the ida nadi, and the pingala nadi. In meditation, the breath coming in at the nostril travels down the ida and pingala nadis to the root chakra where kundalini (spiritual prana) is awakened and then travels up the sushumna nadi to the higher chakras.

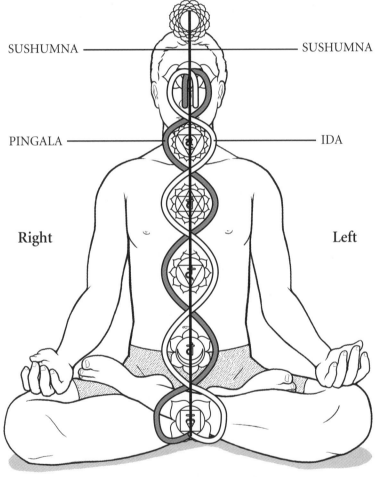

Figure 3: *Yukta Triveni (Repeated)*

The two lotus poles—crown chakra (downward-facing lotus) and root chakra (upward-facing lotus)—connect, the other chakras come into alignment, and the mind calms. As the kundalini rises, it sparks an understanding of the spiritual nature of reality moving us to shift priorities to the spiritual path. Many people think that self-discipline is what keeps people meditating and doing other spiritual practices, but while effort is important, it is kundalini that provides the inclination to put our efforts into spiritual practice.

The term *kundalini* means "coiled like a rope." This energy is typically pictured as a snake coiled in the root chakra and has been referred to as the serpent power. Yoga asanas (poses), prana breathing practices, and mantra practices—body, breath, and sound—also arouse kundalini. As noted above, when you sit in meditation and concentrate on the breath, the kundalini naturally rises up the sushumna to the crown chakra. Some accounts of rising kundalini describe this process as a burst of energy suddenly shooting up the sushumna nadi and producing a big reaction, either positive or negative. There are some dramatic accounts of psychological or physical difficulties that have unfortunately stuck in the popular imagination producing a fear of this energy.

Another reason why kundalini is viewed with trepidation by some in the West is, I believe, a result of the demonization of the unconscious that has been the unintended consequence of some types of psychoanalytic theories that have ascribed innate negative forces to the unconscious. This has contributed to the widespread alienation from the self in the West. Many gurus such as the founder of the Kundalini Research Institute, Yogi Bhajan, have debunked the fear of kundalini by pointing out that the kundalini energy is a part of us. "And what is going to be uncoiled is already in you, it is in dormant power, it is going to uncoil in you. Where danger can be something from outside is put in you then it is dangerous. But already if your system is already built in for that, simply you are not utilizing that energy and you start utilizing that energy, where is the danger?"[4]

I have found both in my own spiritual practice and work with others that the subtle body (chakras, nadis, prana, shakti, and kundalini)

---

4. Yogi Bhajan Lecture Archives, "Kundalini Yoga and Human Radiance," http://fateh.sikhnet.com/sikhnet/articles.nsf, acessed January 1, 2017.

is a user-friendly system. The impetus is toward growth and healing. *Shakti* is concentrated prana that functions as spiritual force or grace. *Kundalini* is the potent shakti energy that abides in the root chakra.

Kundalini is a force that is a natural part of our lives, and if we are not connecting with it, we are not living fully. That is not to say that care is not necessary. You would not attempt to run a marathon without any previous running experience. If you go on a long (days, weeks, or months) retreat, meditating for hours daily without any previous meditation experience, it is possible that you may develop what is called in the East "meditation sickness." When the body and mind are not properly prepared and the prana (chi) rises too quickly, you may experience symptoms such as headaches, dizziness, or stomachaches. The cure is to simply let off of meditating until it goes away. Do *asanas*, eat a healthy diet, and you will ground yourself. If you ever feel unstable psychologically or emotionally while meditating, leave it off and develop a regular yoga practice instead.

Most often kundalini is subtle and the meditator is unaware of it. You will just notice that your attention begins to veer more to spiritual practices and you begin *doing* more of them rather than just reading about them. I think of kundalini as having three stages. The first stage is when it "awakens" and begins to move up the sushumna during meditation, sparking and sustaining our determination to do the practices. The second stage occurs when consistent practice stimulates the heart chakra. Now we are happiest when doing our spiritual practices and discontented if we abandon them. We literally fall in love with spiritual practice. In the third stage, we become connected to the crown chakra and spiritual understanding blooms. Like the lotus, although kundalini rises, it remains firmly planted in the root chakra grounding the higher energies in the moment.

••• EXERCISE: HOW TO MEDITATE •••
USING THREE ACTION STEPS

Take any comfortable seated posture, preferably a cross-legged one. Make sure that your back is straight, your shoulders are down and relaxed, your chin is slightly tilted downwards, your tip of the tongue is relaxed at the point where your upper teeth meet your gums, and your eyes are slightly open with a soft gaze on the floor in front of you. Hold your hands in your lap in the dyana mudra, but with your left palm resting in the right and your thumbs touching each other at your dantian (svadhisthana, pelvic chakra).

Step 1: Concentration on Breath

Concentrate on the breath as it enters and leaves the nostrils. The breathing is gentle and the out breath is always longer than the in breath—about twice as long (e.g., five counts in and ten counts out).

The area between the nostrils and the upper lip, known as the philtrum or infranasal depression, is not associated with a chakra. As we now know, when we focus on a particular chakra, that chakra's consciousness dominates our mind. By focusing attention on the spot where the breath enters and leaves the nostrils, we free our mind from domination by any one chakra's consciousness and we connect with the ida and pingala nadis that come out of the nostrils. Ida and pingala connect back to the root chakra, activating present moment consciousness and awakening kundalini.

Step 2: Mindfulness on the Pelvic Chakra

Be mindful of the point right below the navel where your thumbs touch your body—the pelvic chakra (dantian or hara). This focal point brings the awareness below the solar plexus chakra and helps to calm and center the mind. Remember that mindfulness is not engagement but awareness. When you breathe in, contract this point. When you breathe out, expand it. This is belly breathing and it helps to keep awareness at the pelvic chakra—the center of gravity in the body and the source of power to stay on the spiritual path. Don't concentrate here but rather gently rest your awareness there. Think of it as a centripetal force that pulls the mind toward its center.

Step 3: Mantra

Repeat a phrase in your mind that will help you drop the ego, cut off thinking, and expand the mind. The first part of the phrase is repeated on the inhalation and the second part on the exhalation. Three common Zen phrases are:

In breath	*Out breath*
Just Here	Just Now
Zen Mind	Beginner's Mind
Clear Mind	Don't Know

Let these words float on the breath so that concentration is not disturbed. The words and the breath become one. Just Now cuts off the solar plexus chakra's dash to the future, Beginner's Mind cuts off the solar plexus chakra's ego inflating, and Don't Know establishes a letting-go open consciousness and is an antidote to the solar plexus chakra's "I know."

Overview and Additional Tips

So the three active steps are (1) alert the mind with concentration on the breath as it enters and leaves the nostrils, (2) gain awareness at the pelvic chakra, and (3) repeat phrases that help to focus, open, and clear the mind. Do not try to stop anything from arising or suppressing thoughts and feelings. Instead, think of yourself as not engaging them. You are simply returning to the one-pointed concentration on the breath. A popular teaching is to view thoughts like clouds that come and go, always changing shape, moving, and dissipating.

Six Passive Phases of Meditation

Meditation is a letting-go activity. The passive phases are like gears that shift in the mind, steadily moving us closer and closer to a state of absorption.

- We begin to meditate and the outside world dominates.
- The mind shifts to an inner/outer balance.
- The breath becomes quiet.
- The breath becomes even more subtle.
- The mind settles down.
- Mind energy is concentrated.

Again, these phases require no effort—just persistence with the three action steps: concentration, awareness, and phrases to open the mind. To quiet and concentrate the mind energy, we generally need more than daily short periods of meditation. Retreats with longer periods of sitting allow the mind to settle.

The above is intended as a general road map of the process of meditation—everyone is different and meditation practice should never be judged or compared. Remember that even if you only realize once that your mind has wandered and bring it back to the breath, then you are meditating. There are Zen stories in which someone walking along hears a loud sound and attains sudden realization. At the other end of the extreme it may take someone years of regular practice to let go of distraction and shift the mind to an inner/outer balance.

Do not attach to these phases; they are provided to give you an idea of what to expect—just let go and be persistent with the three action steps. Remember that subtle changes in your outlook and life will happen regardless of where you are in your meditation practice. Where you are in your practice doesn't matter; it is the practice itself that matters. Spiritual growth happens at every point. If you are not ready for meditation, let it go. Everyone is different, just honor where you are—that in itself is growth and healing. However, if you have difficulty with meditation bringing up distressing material, you can always try a short om/lam meditation for five or ten minutes and see if that helps your inner focus without bringing up anything. If you continue to be disturbed, try doing yoga instead and maybe come back to meditation in the future.

••• EXERCISE: OM/LAM TECHNIQUE ••• TO ASSIST WITH MEDITATION

If you are having difficulty with the shift to an inner/outer mind balance, try repeating om/lam (om on the inhale and lam on the exhale) in the mind—this activates the crown and root chakras, creating an energy connection between them by capturing the prana from ida (the sun) and pingala (the moon) nadis and concentrating it in the sushumna nadi connecting these two lotus poles. If you use this om/

lam technique, use it as an aid that you call in from time to time, use briefly, and eventually let go. While it helps to bring the focus within and steady the mind, it also stimulates the subtle body energy, and you want the mind to settle down.

Whenever we sit and begin meditation, the mind is shifting gears. When you concentrate on the breath and decrease distracting thoughts, space opens in the mind for wisdom to arise. The mind is continually settling and opening.

When Pairing Meditation and Traya

After each Traya session, you will feel uplifted and even exhilarated. This comes from *pranothana*—the positive charge of new energy into the subtle body from the release of the samskaras in step 3 (release) and the taking in of new positive prana in step 4 (replace and imprint). The stimulation will usually last for a full day. This helps incentivize us to continue the process. For even though negative material may come up, we are most often left with a markedly uplifted sensation nevertheless.

Because of this, it is important to make sure that the Traya process is separate from your daily meditation. Practicing meditation after Traya will make it difficult to meditate, due to Traya's exhilarating and stimulating pranothana effect. I don't mean that you will be thinking more, but that the inner subtle body energy is "bubbling" and the mind energy cannot settle. To ensure you are getting the full benefits of your meditation practice, remember to first meditate and do Traya at some point after.

Yoga and the Chakras

Yoga cleanses both the mind and body of toxins via the asanas, breathing, and various other practices. Traya practice, with its historical connection to Tantra and its focus on purification of the mind, adds yet another tool. Yoga means unity. The solar plexus chakra separates mind, body, and spirit, so here the goal is also to decrease that separation. In Pantanjali's *Yoga Sutras* (written before 400 CE) he states,

"The restraint of the modifications of the mind-stuff is yoga." [5] Physical asanas help to free us from the solar plexus chakra tendency to be in our heads by connecting us with our bodies (root chakra), and if done mindfully, can be a moving meditation. If we watch our minds during our yoga practice, we see that our "like-don't like" mind will appear when we approach a difficult, strenuous posture or one that is difficult for our body. If we just focus on our breathing and posture, we have a more engaged experience.

The balance poses help us see how inattention interferes with the moment connection. If you are in tree pose, for example, and you lose your focus and start thinking about something else, you lose your balance. In life we can lose our balance if we do not pay attention.

The term *asana* means seat and represents the root of the lotus— our connection to our body and the earth. Energy moving to higher chakras must be countered by grounding in the body. Just as yoga asanas are designed to act on specific parts of the body, they also stimulate the subtle body in both general and specific ways by dispersing prana throughout the subtle body, rather than being congested at the solar plexus—a common tendency.

"Asanas and prana are designed to purify the nadis, for when they are blocked prana cannot flow freely and poor health results." [6]

Asanas were developed specifically for this purpose—to help us connect with the body to help calm and clear the mind for meditation practice and to keep the body strong and flexible so that we can persist in meditation. Manifestation requires that both the crown chakra and the root chakra are strong and engaged. Yoga constantly charges the root chakra and stimulates all of them.

In your yoga practice, be sure to include at least one asana from each of the main pose categories: standing, sitting, forward bending,

5. Sri Swami Satchidananda, *The Yoga Sutras of Pantanjali: Translation and Commentary by Sri Swami Satchidananda* (Buckingham, VA: Integral Yoga Publications, 2008), 3.

6. Lucy Lidell, Narayani, and Giris Rabinovitch, *The Sivananda Companion to Yoga: A Complete Guide to the Physical Postures, Breathing exercises, Diet, Relaxation and Meditation Techniques of Yoga* (New York: Simon and Schuster, 2000), 68.

backward bending, side bending, balance poses, inversions, and twists so that prana moves throughout the entire body. This flowing prana stimulates all of the chakras but especially the root chakra and, therefore, kundalini. Our desire for further spiritual practice is sparked and we are firmly established in the lotus energy (spiritual prana).

The body is the manifestation of the moment as all bodily sensations are experienced right now. With asanas we mobilize the energies of the body to tame the mind. The body follows the mind so it is important to do yoga so we can turn it around and have the mind follow the body and become "body full." Yoga is not a "workout," it is a "work-in." Mind-body awareness produces mind-body intelligence. Let the mind follow the body in yoga and then there will be more balance and the mind can then follow the body to meditation practice and more yoga. With experience, this connection reduces the distracting influence of our thoughts.

In meditation we keep our body still so our mind will follow and become still. It is through the body that we connect to ourselves and to the spiritual senses; the sense of grounding, connection, and compassion, these are in the body. Our bodies let us know when we are going in the right or wrong direction. It is important to be firmly established in our body, inhabiting it fully and grounded in the moment in order for spiritual growth, our blooming lotus, to flourish.

As noted, all asanas impact the subtle body and the root chakra in particular as this is where physical body consciousness resides. The following are a few examples of asanas that impact each of the seven primary chakras specifically. Note that the chakras open in both the front and the back of the body. *Salambasana*, for example, stimulates the pelvic chakra in the lower back.

Crown chakra: Head stand (sirsasana) or any inversion—this sets the crown chakra "spinning" in search for universal connection, like a computer searching for the internet connection.

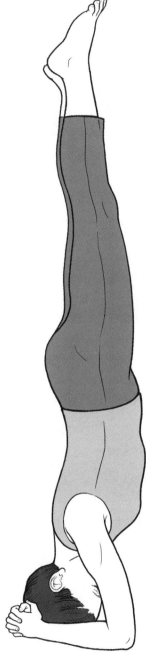

Figure 4A: sirsasana

Third eye chakra: Head to knee pose (janu sirsasana), half-tortoise (ardha-kurmasana) and yoga seal (yoga mudrasana)

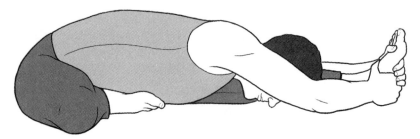

Figure 4B: janu sirsasana

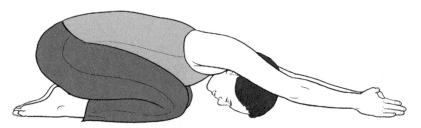

Figure 4C: ardha kurmasana

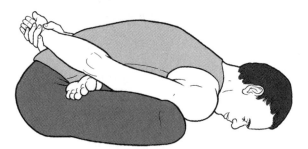

Figure 4D: yoga mudrasana

Throat chakra: Shoulder stand (sarvangasana) and fish pose (matsyasana)

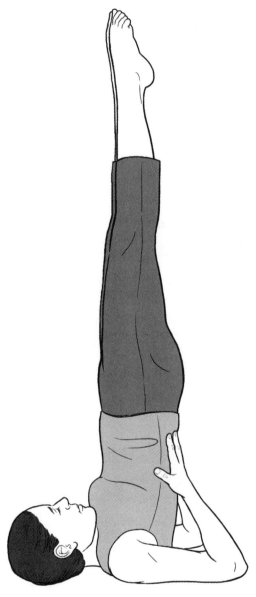

Figure 4E: sarvangasana

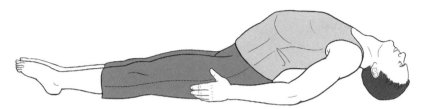

Figure 4F: matsyasana

Heart chakra: Camel (ustrasana) and other backward bending poses

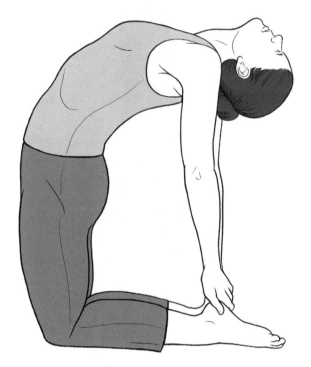

Figure 4G: ustrasana

Solar plexus chakra: Bow pose (dhanurasana), seated twist (ardha-matsyendrasana)

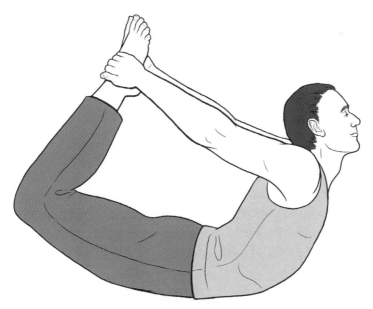

Figure 4H: dhanurasana

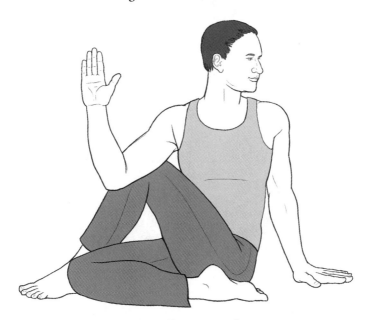

Figure 4I: ardha matsyendrasana

Pelvic chakra: Locust pose (salabhasana) and all balance poses

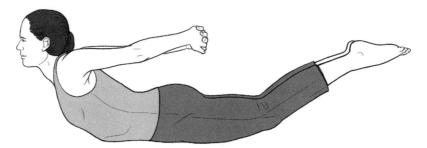

Figure 4J: salabhasana

Root chakra: All asanas, especially garland (malasana) seated poses and inversions. Inverted positions stimulate this chakra and set it searching for the earth connection. Again, think of a computer searching for a Wi-Fi connection.

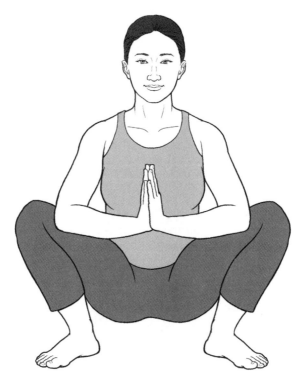

Figure 4K: malasana

Chanting lower chakra seed sounds helps connect with asanas. For example, when doing balancing standing poses, chant vam (the pelvic chakra bija) either out loud or silently. This helps to keep attention at the pelvic chakra and enables one to stay in the pose longer because it holds our center of gravity. It is helpful to use the root chakra seed sound lam when in a pose that stretches the leg and/or lower back muscles. Focus on the tightness and chant lam in your mind and this helps to both loosen the muscles and to strengthen the lower body connection. Chanting at the beginning of the class stimulates the subtle body so that the asanas can more readily move prana throughout the nadis. The Hari Om mantra, particularly, stimulates the chakras and is said to remove suffering.

••• EXERCISE: CHAKRA STIMULATING ••• YOGA FLOW

If you have a regular practice and are familiar with these poses, try a short home practice to stimulate each chakra in turn. Focus your attention on breathing at the chakra and repeat the bija silently or aloud while in the pose:

- Sit in a cross-legged posture and chant Hari Om, Hari Om, Hari, Hari, Hari Om several times. Then:
- In garland pose (malasana), focus at the root chakra and repeat the bija lam.
- In locust pose (salabhasana), focus at the pelvic center and repeat the bija vam.
- In bow pose (dhanurasana), focus at the solar plexus and repeat its bija ram.
- In camel pose (ustrasana), focus at the center of the chest and repeat yam.
- In shoulder stand (sarvangasana), focus at the center of the neck and repeat ham.

- In fish pose (matsyasana), focus at the center of the neck and repeat ham.
- In head to knee pose (janu sirsasana), focus at the third eye and repeat hum.
- In half tortoise pose (ardha kurmasana), focus at the third eye and repeat hum.
- In head stand (sirsasana), focus on the crown and repeat om.
- Then in yogic seal (yoga mudrasana), seal the energies within.

If you like the flow of vinyasa, you can add a chaturanga (low plank, upward dog, and downward dog) between each pose. Finish with savasana and notice the stimulated subtle body energy as you relax.

Gunas

The Three Gunas, or sets of qualities—sattva (light, consciousness), rajas (action, attachment), and tamas (heavy, dark)—are found both throughout nature and in human consciousness. The chakras have varying amounts of each of these qualities—the higher chakras, third eye and crown, are predominately sattvic, the solar plexus chakra (diaphragm) is predominately rajasic, and the lowest, root chakra, is predominantly tamasic. Yoga helps us to balance the mind by balancing these qualities. When we focus on the physical body in yoga, tamas, or grounding, is increased and the restlessness and distraction of the rajasic solar plexus chakra that is so common in our modern society is decreased.

Yoga therapists can apply Traya to help balance the gunas. There are also specific yoga therapy protocols using Traya to address stress, fear, worry, addictions, codependence, and insomnia.

Pranayama (yogic breathing) and chanting lift the energy to the higher chakras and increase sattvic qualities in our minds—peace, harmony, and spirit. Practicing both meditation and yoga balances the energy between the two lotus poles: meditation activates the crown chakra and yoga activates the root chakra. When we heal the higher chakras, we enter the realm of spiritual focus, insight, and power; and our Inner Lotus, firmly planted in the root chakra, is then ready to fully bloom into the Lotus of Full Potential.

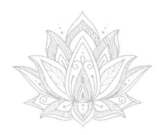

Chapter 5

THE STAGES OF CHANGE THROUGH THE TRAYA PROCESS

Traya is a gentle and organic process that can be likened to a soothing compress on an infected wound—samskaras are gently surfaced and, if we are persistent, the wound heals, our bodies get stronger, and our minds more peaceful and positive. We are recovering the self that had been shut out by the pain body. If your pain body is weak, these stages will not all apply to you as they address recovery from a significant pain body, nevertheless, you may see yourself in some of the topics discussed. Stage one begins the deconstruction of the pain body, stage two is the transitional phase, stage three is reconstructing the true body, and stage four is transformation. Stage four, transformation, applies to all.

The length of time you'll spend in each of these stages depends on how many samskaras you have in your chakras, how long they have been there, the intensity of the samskaras, what your goals are, and, most importantly, your dedication to the process. A regular meditation and yoga practice will help you to stay grounded and centered. I encourage you to continue working as you reach your goal(s), for there is much to be gained by completing the entire process of change.

Stage One: Deconstructing the Pain Body

Up to this point we have been reacting to the pain body and trying to distract ourselves from the pain of its grip. Now we must engage the subtle body and activate the change process.

Awakening the Subtle Body

In this beginning stage, our minds are full of worries and negative thoughts. The solar plexus chakra's judging energy may tell us that Traya is not going to work. We don't yet understand the impact of different types of experiences and when samskaras from childhood rejection by a friend or a negative and a disapproving parental face arise, we think, "Oh why haven't I gotten over that?" Or the process seems so simple we think, "Can this really work?"

We may have "big T" Traumas that come up over and over again and we wonder why they keep coming up in different chakras. "Big T" Traumas deposit samskaras in various chakras as they are dissonant at every level. Even "small t" traumas may repeatedly come up. For example, many are surprised to find that being left alone often as a child even if there was an adult in the house has a significant impact and will come up at various chakras—at the solar plexus because it contributes to a sense of separateness and isolation; at the heart because the disengagement makes one feel unwanted; at the throat because there is no one to talk to; and perhaps at other chakras also.

In order to build confidence in Traya, I often ask beginners to work with either a solar plexus, pelvic, or throat chakra issue. Focus on it until it disappears. Then you know that anything and everything can change. I see the entire Traya process as one of coming out of hiding and blooming fully within the Lotus of Full Potential.

The Truth of Truth

We begin to see how the mind resonates with truth. No one can give us the truth. It must come from within. We begin to trust our own mind. Again, those in the grip of the "rational" mind find it difficult to give the inner world its due. This is why I almost always first focus on the solar plexus chakra—to relax its hold and open the mind.

Self-Understanding

Most of us have a one-dimensional view of our past. Traya allows us to fill in the picture. As we begin to understand ourselves better, we start to forgive ourselves and let go of guilt or self-condemnation.

Shifts in the Mind and Relief Begins

As issues such as fear decrease, we notice that we respond in ways we weren't anticipating or planning. One twenty-year-old was surprised when, after some work with the throat chakra, he observed himself doing something he was never able to do before. Chad's father often behaved angrily toward him and chastised him if he protested. His mother corrected him if he responded to his father. This was frustrating for Chad but he didn't want to fight with his mother too. One day, as this familiar scenario was playing out, he said to his mother, "Why do you always take his side and never see my side?" He later told me, "I surprised myself, the words just came out of my mouth—I wasn't even thinking about it." This was the beginning of his coming out of hiding and taking up vocal space.

Stage Two: Transitioning

Space in the Mind and Rise of the Positive

There is now more space in the mind for positive thoughts to come through and counter the negative ones. I recognize this stage when I begin to hear statements like the following:

"When I was feeling sad, I said to myself, 'This will pass. It won't last because it never lasted before.'"

"Maybe [life] is an experiment and I am privileged to be here— just go with it."

"I realize that if he doesn't choose me, it has nothing to do with who I am."

Further Shifts—Recognition of Patterns

As we continue to experience relief, we see more clearly the connections between our experiences and repetitive patterns playing out over and over in our lives despite our determination to change. We felt like puppets controlled by samskaric strings, pulled by the pain body, reprising scenes from the past. When we are not pulled as strongly to feel or behave in a familiar way, this can be slightly disorienting. Yet it is surprising how quickly we adapt to these changes. Some examples of these types of shifts are:

Moira felt more self-assured and powerful, which to her, "feels odd because I see someone I don't fully recognize and I am still learning to own it."

Aimee reports that she no longer feels swept away by big emotions. Anger came and she sat with it and started to explore it and it dissipated.

Raina noticed that she is no longer taking things so personally. "I realize it is about them and not me. This is so clear yet I never saw it before. It is changing the way that I inhabit my life."

Lorna reported that she has noticed that she is not as affected by what others do or not do. "I was not invited to a coworker's wedding and someone else in the office was. I would have been devastated before."

Inner/Outer Connection

There is a saying in Zen, "Everything is created by mind alone." In chapter 8 we will see how the solar plexus chakra imposes a structure on the world, creating subject and object, time and space, the ten directions, etc. That is one way that the mind creates our reality and there is another way. Prana is active in our lives and the outside world complies with the state of our chakras. A strong pain body makes problems, and when it weakens, problems disappear and positive situations appear. The subtle body has power—the power to create our reality. The distinction between inside and outside is more permeable than we realize. Some of it is obvious and some is not. It is obvious that if we have anger, our relationships will suffer because we will put people off. Some of this is very subtle and takes time to see.

As these repetitive situations appear again, samskaras having already been reduced, there is less drama and intensity. For example, if you had a rigidly controlling parent, you may attract a controlling boss but he or she won't be as draconian. Now these patterns are clear and we can turn them into healing opportunities. As we face them without fear and get a positive result, our healing is affirmed and reinforced. We see that our mind creates our reality by actually drawing people and situations to us. As habitual patterns dissipate, liberated prana mobilizes the outside world to align with our new positive outlook and attitude. Positive people and situations are attracted to us and we to them. The beauty of the mind amazes us and we find that we are beginning to comprehend it.

Relationships Improve

As we continue to open, more information surfaces, our insight grows, and we develop a trusting relationship with our deep mind. We do not question, "Am I making this up?" or "Did I put that there?" when memories come up. We pay attention to what makes us feel better and stop doing the things that don't make us feel good. Charles came in and reported, "I have stopped watching porn. I want to do things that make me feel better rather than being compulsive."

This self-care includes how we behave with other people. I saw this with Raina, who presented herself as someone wise but tough in her dealings with others. She said, when describing a situation with a supervisor, "In the past, my 'fuck you' attitude just came out—I had to carry conflict within me instead of with other people and I never thought of the effect on me. Now I think of how will I feel."

We begin to see clearly the roles that we play with people and begin to let go of them. It was becoming clear to Sheryl that her spiritual teacher served as a negative parental stand-in. He would often give her "the silent treatment," as did her mother, or he would overlook her contributions to the group while praising others for theirs. He would highlight others' birthdays and coldly ignore hers. "He is my mother in male form." Yet she was not able to stop attending the group and reacting to this teacher. There is a saying attributed to the Buddha: "Your worst enemy is your best teacher." We don't have to stay in a relationship with someone who is pushing our samskaric buttons, but if the pull is too strong to cut, then it is good to have the perspective that it is helping us heal by bringing up the samskaras from the past that create this strong attraction and dark places of vulnerability so that we can finally see them, heal them, and move on.

After a session working with the third eye chakra, Sheryl realized that she accepted this behavior because she believed that she was bad and deserved this type of treatment, and released the associated samskaras. She also had the insight that there was a strong negative dynamic between both of them that activated pain body material in each. She realized that she contributed to people treating her badly—because of her belief that she was bad. This clear perception replaced her denial, gave her some distance from the experiences and also a newfound sense of control. In her struggle with letting go of this teacher, the universe provided a nudge. She ran into someone who had left this same group and this person told her of difficulties with this same teacher, whom she saw as "supremely egotistical." The evidence and support was mounting and she was soon able to let go of the teacher and stop attending the group.

We can activate our environments both to attract those who will reenact our past and also, when enough samskaras have been released, to attract those who will help us make a necessary change. From this position of strength, we see that if there is negativity in relationships with other people, we must first look to see if there is something inside of us that needs to be cleared.

Traya is a self-reflective process in which we take responsibility for our relationships in a non-blaming way because we now understand the power of samskaric residue in the mind. We feel more comfortable with people and we stop acting on any remaining negativity. Life becomes easier and flows more smoothly. Sara once said, "I am less defended and more out there. I have fewer sore spots."

As we change we find more joy from simple contact without expectations. We also see how others' pain bodies impacted their relationships and have compassion for their suffering too. As our relationship with both ourselves and others improves, we are even more motivated to continue growing.

Low heart chakra energy in particular can move us to cling to the wrong people. Feeling so empty inside, we need a people fix, so we seek out people even if they are not the best company for us. There is a point in this process for many who have surrounded themselves with inappropriate people, to take a step back and stop engaging so readily with them. We don't completely drop them but they somehow move from the foreground to the background of our lives as we allow more positive relationships to come in. This takes trust and the patience to tolerate a period less full of people. We eventually see that it was impossible to be close to these people and we needed it that way because we, also, were afraid of closeness.

Dreams

When we start to understand the messages of our dreams and then follow up with the Traya work, the psyche feels heard and understood and more dreams come through. Dreams are the psyche's way of pointing to material that it wants expunged now, and we must always honor the psyche. In this and the next phase, dreamwork takes a more active role, as we are more connected to ourselves and the psyche responds to that.

Disillusion—Fear It Won't Change

The heart sometimes feels like it takes longer to heal than the other chakras as it doesn't usually exhibit step-by-step improvements as the others do. The steadily decreasing fear in the solar plexus chakra and the steadily improving communication in the throat chakra, for example, urge us to keep doing Traya. The heart chakra will sometimes feel worse until it suddenly shifts to positive. So factors like length of time required, its state of hopelessness and distrust when samskaric, and the lack of evidence that it is getting better, until it does, can present a challenge. Don't give up. Positive change gained from healing other chakras can be used as evidence that persistence produces rewards. When the positive attributes of a healthy heart chakra appear—particularly the switch from a sense of sadness and emptiness to fullness, buoyancy, confidence, and love of self and life, one feels an abiding sense of support from the universe.

Resistance—Fear It Will Change

This is a transformative process and letting go of the familiar can generate some resistance even when we can see clearly that what we hold on to causes us pain. Our suffering can sometimes feel like a wrap or a cloak and we can be hesitant to let it go for we do not yet know what will take its place or how to be in the world without it. Paradoxically, it is in this transitional stage when positive changes are happening and one sees the real possibility of freedom from the pain body and all that it brings with it, that one may hesitate. This is usually related to fear of the unknown and identification with suffering. We have the wrong belief that the pain body is an essential part of our identity. If we have related to others through negative bickering or to life through our sadness, we are afraid to let it go for fear of the potential loss of that connection. We do not yet fully trust that as we step unencumbered into life we will be met generously and supportingly. Sometimes in my workshops people will say, "But that is part of what makes me who I am." I always respond that this is an illusion. Suffering is keeping you from knowing who you are and what you are capable of. One woman spoke of the son of a Holocaust survivor she knows who didn't want to give up his anger. I responded that underneath anger there is sadness and vulnerability. Anger is a more active energy that allows him to keep from sinking into his pain. I reminded her that any negativity in us impacts both self and other. We may think that our anger is protecting us, but as the saying goes, "Holding on to anger is like picking up a hot rock to throw at another. We are the ones that get burned." Those close to us are impacted also, for negativity in our hearts disconnects us from them.

Small pain body issues resolve quickly. A large one takes time and is a step-by-step process usually taking several years, depending on how much there is to unravel. Of course, even if you have a large pain body, if you do Traya every day, change will come much quicker. Regardless of how long to attain your goals, change is always happening every time you do the Traya work. Over time, we learn to trust that each time we let go of negative there is not emptiness but positive that takes its place. There is an inner stability and balance that comes with healing the solar plexus chakra and this gives us the determination to keep going.

Sometimes we need encouragement. One of the ways the Inner Teacher encourages us is in the positive imprint part of the Traya work when you are bringing in light (step 4). Sheila received the message, "We are happy you are doing this work." Even though the Inner Teacher may speak to us many times, at this stage we may not yet fully trust it. Hold on to the positive messages you receive—it is coming from somewhere very important.

As the relationship with the Inner Teacher strengthens, trust grows and resistance disappears. In Hinduism, the god Shiva in the form of Nataraja represents liberation from the fear of change. He is depicted dancing within a ring of fire, symbolizing the burning up of old perspectives. His lower right hand is in the *abhaya* mudra, reminding us to fear not. Chanting the mantra *om namah shivaya*, especially while in this transition phase is beneficial, as the five elements present in the chakras (earth, water, fire, air, and ether) are invoked, while om stimulates the higher chakras.

Stage Three: Liberating the True Body
The following are signals that this stage has been reached.

Themes Appear
In the first stages of Traya work, negative memories and patterns predominate. In this stage, themes too appear along with a wider perspective. For example, in previous stages, Katarina's bullying memories related to her personal life and now the larger theme of "man's inhumanity to man" appears.

Things Lacking Appear
As the pain body diminishes, the healthy aspects of the chakras strengthen and we find our:

- Voice
- Self-esteem
- Confidence and motivation
- Boundaries
- Grounding
- Drive
- Accomplishment
- Joy and enthusiasm
- Insight

We see that happiness is an inside job and doesn't come from outside things. Francine shared, "My default mode is now happy. I wake up happy. I have regained my connection to the part of my childhood that was happy."

Now, we see ourselves more clearly and experience life more fully. Our energy is now in sync with the flow of life, no longer trying to make things happen but letting everything grow up around us while standing in our authenticity.

Some Examples of People in This Stage

One of Francine's core issues was feeling unsupported, particularly at work. "Now I am more focused on all of those supporting me, rather than on who is not." She is in the same company with the same people but her experience of it is different. "I am now working on degrees of wellness—polishing the wellness. Sometimes I can't believe I am so happy and I am afraid that I will lose it."

Jim had always felt squeezed financially with an "existential sense of dread." He now feels the heart chakra's sense of abundance. He gives generously, lives well, and always has enough. He would sometimes say, "I don't know how this happened. My relationship to money is completely different."

Sheryl once said, "I am doing exactly what I want to do. My heart can be itself. I feel more warmth and light. I have things to look forward to."

Perhaps Sheryl, Jim, and Francine still have more work to do, but they are all having new healthier experiences they never had before, all the while building a secure foundation that supports their continued change and growth.

Shift in Locus of Influence

When we occupy ourselves more fully, the "locus of influence" naturally switches from external to internal and we stop looking outside for approval, answers, or validation, I know someone is in this stage when I hear something like this: *"I am now able to take my head out of the equation and go with what really feels right."*

We see how the pain body interfered with intuitive signals. Ideas and "wants" had more focus and weight than intuition and experience. Now decisions are inner-influenced and the genuine needs of the self take precedence. When Bob reached this stage, he said, "I am not invisible to myself anymore."

Tela, a young and attractive woman in her thirties, had a tendency to get involved with men who weren't that into her. Although she lived in New York City, she had met a man on a trip to Miami where she traveled regularly on business and had a "crush" on him. He was sending clear signals that his interest was primarily sexual by not contacting her when she was home in New York City. Her denial energy in the third eye chakra kept her interested in him, but she was able to state, "I realize that the tightness in the stomach I feel when with Charles is a warning to not go too fast or to not go forward at all." Her locus of influence has shifted.

Inner Compass

The third eye, heart, and the solar plexus chakras help us know our purpose and direction. In the heart we will feel a sense of fullness when heading in the right direction (pursuing our heart's true desire) and in the solar plexus we feel a sense of contraction when we are not (as with Tela)—the third eye chakra is more subtle and we may not feel it, but it is influencing us nevertheless. These are the arrows on our inner compass helping us maneuver through life. It is something like aligning with the *Tao*, the flow of life. There are currents that are flowing in the direction that we need to go. It doesn't mean that following the positive energy is effortless. Reaching goals involves work and effort. It just means that we let go and trust that following our inner guidance is the most effective route.

Inner Teacher

As the positive energy increases, we can feel the presence of the Inner Teacher more, as its voice comes through loud and clear. Now we know with confidence and certainty that we can never be alone again, for it is there whenever we seek it out. When we finish meditating and ask, "What do I need to know today?" it responds clearly with advice such as "Stay in the moment."

Increased Focus on Passion

As the locus of influence shifts to internal, our focus shifts to our purpose. Samskaric distractions, denial, fear, and procrastination prevented us from pursuing goals close to our heart—our true work. Ellen, now freed of her panic attacks, stated, "I am so happy to be concerned about real things (where work life is going) rather than how I feel."

There is an increase in creative energy and focus on what we need to express in our own unique way. On what is truly worth an investment of our time and energy. It is as if something in us is geared toward the achievement of our true purpose, and when we are off course, the psyche warns us. If we pay attention, we get back on course and stay there.

Coming Out of Hiding

Traya is essentially a process of coming out of hiding and living authentically. We were hiding both from others and ourselves. When we heal the three "hiding" chakras in particular, we are more active in the world—doing energy in the root chakra, engagement energy in the solar plexus chakra, and "showing ourselves" energy in the throat chakra all move us to participate fully.

Sara hid behind a markedly cheery and smiley false persona for as long as she could remember. She went to a wedding of a good friend and reported: "I had another friend watch for my 'false persona.' I had a blast and never fell into that. That was completely new for me."

Ellen, who began the Traya process with a high level of fear, came in and at this point stated, "I am not anxious anymore for no reason. I feel more comfortable with strangers—more like myself. It is a relief to feel so much more comfortable in all types of social situations."

Francine said, "I now see that the positive energy serves as my protection—it is my Jedi sword. Defenses I built up before were actually in my way instead of protecting me." Now, living in a positive energy field and feeling fully supported by the universe, we participate more fully.

Emotional Growth and Integration

It is in this reconstruction stage that we fully reclaim our emotions. Self-esteem moves us to acknowledge the importance of all of our feelings.

Before the Traya work, Sara didn't have access to her anger as her emotional energy was blocked in the pelvic chakra. "I now have deep emotions like other people. Previously, I only felt sad, awkward, or uncomfortable." We now enter a deeper level of healing—more substantive and lingering. We become aware of more subtle states of being. She said, "I feel like I am more in my own life. I have been feeling more centered lately so I notice more when I am not there."

Gloria once said, "I had been deeply hurt and invisible to myself. I am giving myself permission to be in the pain and hurt. I am sitting with it whereas before I didn't even know about it."

Children learn to understand their feelings by integrating them with their experience. As we grow we learn to understand why we feel certain ways at certain times and start to own those feelings. We learn to avoid people or situations that don't feel good. When those situations are in the home or other parts of the environment that we can't avoid, however, we cope by repressing feelings and fail to learn these crucial lessons. If our parents were disconnected from their feelings, we then do the same. If our feelings are not respected by others, then we don't respect them either. Perhaps there was blame or criticism for feeling certain ways.

In this stage emotional integration is well on its way and now we understand the material we have been surfacing and the themes that we have been working with on an emotional level. We may surprise ourselves by crying in a situation we wouldn't have before. Perhaps we are happy for someone and we shed a tear of happiness or a movie makes us cry where it wouldn't have before. Or the opposite happens—if we were overemotional, our emotions now come into balance. Sometimes feelings will arise while meditating and we get in touch with some sadness we hadn't connected with before. We are becoming completely human and emotions are an important part of us.

Balance

By healing the solar plexus chakra, we are balancing the right brain and the left brain. The mind is now less reactive. We are living deeper in the ocean of our own lives and less on the surface, so there is less fluctuation and turbulence. There is a sense of lightness and life flows with ease. When problems do come, the mind stays steady and we take a balanced approach to solving them. We have achieved equanimity. No more extreme highs and lows.

Joy in Little Things

At this stage one carries a sense of joie de vivre. We find joy in life from simple contact with nature and with other people. We are comforted with the knowledge that we are part of something larger and know that the grass is greenest beneath our own feet; we feel a sense of gratitude just for being alive. We slow down, are more present, and often focus on improving our surroundings. Judith reported, "I am taking delight in every detail of my apartment where as before it was a wreck. I hadn't slept in my bedroom for two years and now I am fixing it all up."

Things Work Out

When we have reached the reconstruction stage, we understand more fully how Traya works. With positive-thinking and self-help strategies, there is an attempt to bring about a desired change by imagining that it has already occurred in one's life. "I now have all the money I need" or "I now have the relationship that I want," for example. Believing that something is true makes it true. With Traya, on the other hand, the change happens and then the belief has to catch up. One of the things that we notice is that somehow things generally work out the way that we want them as the positive attributes of the chakras are creating situations resonant with them. The right situations and the right people come to us at the right time. We just need to do the groundwork to be prepared to meet these opportunities when they appear. We feel a sense of grace and synchronicity. Over time we start to believe that this will continue. Sheryl exclaimed one day, "I have a constant feeling of the goodness of the universe and ease of everything."

Impact on the Physical Body

Traya is a mind–body practice, as the chakras connect with both mind and body. This mind–body connection becomes clear when we examine a symptom such as anxiety that has defined chemical markers and can be mitigated with pharmaceutical drugs. The hormones cortisol and adrenaline are produced by fear. As fear and worry decrease, these hormones come into a healthier balance. Neurotransmitters such as serotonin and endorphins that produce a sense of well-being are elevated as the heart chakra heals. When our mind is balanced we are no longer reactive to external stressors. We no longer live in fight-or-flight mode or carry stress that is well known to have debilitating effects on the body. In my practice over the years, I too noticed that people who get along in life not dealing with their significant samskaras often have physical issues to deal with. If we ignore the mind, then the body gets hit and often hit hard. How does this happen? Each chakra regulates energy flow through its associated area of the body. Each primary chakra is also related to one of the endocrine glands. For example, the heart chakra is located near the thymus gland that regulates our immune system. As you can see from the following illustration, the chakras are located in the same general vicinity as the endocrine glands.

Traya supports physical health by purifying the system and allowing all of the five pranas to work unimpeded. The vibrational field that vitalizes the physical body is raised and we become physically stronger.

Physical tension can remain in the body even when the tense situation has long passed. Just as we carry the memory of the experience, we also carry the physicality of the experience. In other words, the mind tension has been healed with Traya but the body still holds some of it. Body tension energy is usually carried in the solar plexus and the letting go (*mukta*) chakras, and this must also be released to completely relax the body.

When a chakra is weak, there may be physical problems in physical organs in the general area of the chakra. For example, Violet's bowels were severely impacted. We worked with the root chakra, which is related to the downward flowing elimination energy of apana prana. Memories of disagreements and confrontations in her childhood environment and in her current life where she is fighting with her husband surfaced. We know that these types of memories create samskaras related to feeling unsafe in the physical environment. Her Diagnostic Scene from Nature was of a snowy night revealing significant blockages in the root chakra. The root chakra is solid earth energy and we do not want any form of water there. We continued to focus on the root chakra, and the impaction cleared up and she noticed a marked change for the better in her daily bowel movements.

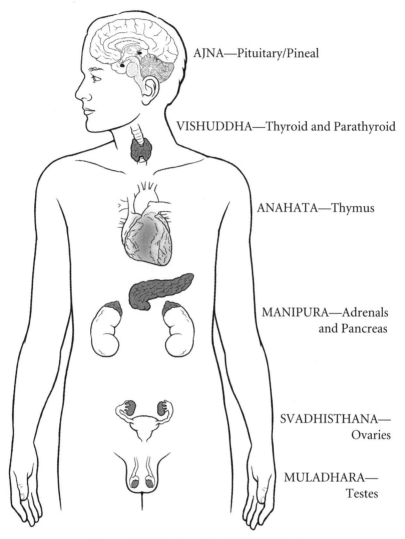

AJNA—Pituitary/Pineal

VISHUDDHA—Thyroid and Parathyroid

ANAHATA—Thymus

MANIPURA—Adrenals
and Pancreas

SVADHISTHANA—
Ovaries

MULADHARA—
Testes

Figure 5: Endocrine Gland Chakra Overlay

If you have a physical ailment, in addition to obtaining the appropriate medical treatment for it, work with it energetically so as to aid and speed the healing process. You can do this by focusing on the chakra in that part of the body and following the same Traya process that is used for removing mind samskaras. For example, problems with the thyroid would be associated with the throat chakra. If in the chest, arms, or hands, the heart and the associated Tertiary chakras in the palms of the hands and elbow crook; if in the legs or feet, the root chakra and the associated Tertiary chakras in the soles of the feet and behind the knees.

Physical injuries (including surgeries) also impact the chakras and produce samskaras—these should be released also as a memory in the nearest chakra. For example, gall bladder surgery released from the solar plexus, or a piece of wood falling on top of the head from the crown chakra, etc.

As more energy becomes available for life it wants to be expressed ,and one of the ways is in the joy of exercise because it gives us a wonderful feeling. We no longer need willpower to do things that are good for us.

As we remove toxins from the chakras, the five elements of earth, water, fire, air, and ether come into balance and strengthen the forces that animate, support, and nourish the mind and body. When we are fully embodied, we can no longer engage in harmful practices such as overeating, over-drinking, or over-exercising. We do not ignore subtle bodily messages until they become a health issue. We notice how good it feels to eat good food, so we stick with the good stuff.

Improvement encourages us to keep going. Integrating meditation and yoga further supports the Lotus of Full Potential within each of us.

Stage Four: Transformation

All spiritual solutions lead back to the self. All genuine teachers point you in the direction of you. Throughout the Traya process we have been balancing the ego, dropping our false personas, and healing the mind of negativity. Many of us have a tendency to overlook spirit in our daily lives except in times of crisis. Jonathan Franzen addresses this in his *New Yorker* essay "Farther Away" (speaking of Robinson Crusoe):

Robinson finds God on the island, and he turns to Him repeatedly in moments of crisis, praying for deliverance and ecstatically thanking Him for providing the means of it. And yet, as soon as each crisis has passed, he reverts to his practical self and forgets about God; by the end of the book, he seems to have been saved more by his own industry and ingenuity than by Providence.[7]

True intimacy with the self requires consistent spiritual attention and practice.

Spiritual Practice and the Chakras

In chapter 1, I presented the concept of two minds—the surface and the deep mind—and we saw that the chakras are the programs that operate or influence these minds. Meditation reveals that there is yet another mind—the mind that mirrors our true nature. It is beyond the chakras because it is the mind that can never be diminished or soiled in any way. Samskaras cannot touch it—they can only distract us from it. It is the clear mind, or our true nature, that we connect with in meditation. Its messenger is our Inner Teacher. It is there regardless of the presence or absence of the pain body.

I remember when I was young and working in a job that dragged me down. I went out to lunch and was feeling very lost and in despair. I went into a bookstore and picked up a book, *The Yoga Sutras of Patanjali*, and suddenly my despair was lifted. This powerful sense came over me that my path, somehow, led in this direction. It was a truly spiritual experience despite the fact that I was chock-full of samskaras. This was but a glimpse, although a powerful one, of my higher self piercing through my despair and giving me a message—although, at the time, I had no idea what it meant. In reading the actual book, I found it very difficult to understand or take in the teachings as my mind was so scattered. Yet, I had a powerful sense of connecting with

7. Jonathan Franzen, "Farther Away," *The New Yorker*, April 18, 2011, https://www.newyorker.com/magazine/2011/04/18/farther-away-jonathan-franzen, accessed January 1, 2016.

something bigger than me. I include this example to point out that this "last" stage of transformation is for everyone, regardless of where they are in the Traya process.

If we are spiritual beings, why is it so much of a struggle to stay engaged with the moment and with spirit? We have healed the solar plexus samskaric afflictions such as fear, worry, and disengagement and now we need to conquer the more subtle spiritual afflictions. The three kleshas of ignorance, attachment, and aversion, known also as the three poisons in Buddhism, remain for us to deal with. It is the solar plexus chakra's nature, even when it is free of samskaras, to make the self-centered "I" and to make "I want" and "I don't want"—grasping and aversion. And this is what keeps us trapped in ignorance. This is what the Buddha put forth as the Second Noble Truth, identifying the basic cause of suffering in life—grasping for things outside of ourselves. "The essence of all Buddha's teachings is aimed at countering our grasping at a sense of self and at self-cherishing thoughts."[8] From a Christian perspective: "If you go out, God will come in."[9]

So escape from the solar plexus chakra's grip on the mind is the foundation of the spiritual quest. When this grip is loosened, the "spiritual" chakras—the crown (universal consciousness), the heart (love, connection, compassion), and the root (in the moment)—are energized. Both meditation and yoga loosen the solar plexus chakra's grip, balance the energies, and bring the chakras into alignment so that we can become sensitive to the subtler sattvic qualities of life and nature and do not lose interest in our spiritual path.

8. The Dalai Lama, *A Profound Mind: Cultivating Wisdom in Everyday Life*, ed. Nicholas Vreeland (New York: Harmony Books, 2011), 127.

9. Seung Sahn, *The Whole World Is A Single Flower: 365 Koans for Everyday Life*, (Rutland, Vermont: Charles E. Tuttle, 2011), 56.

Six Categories of Mind Suffering

Without a regular meditation practice, we still may be drawn in by these six categories of spiritual suffering created even in a healthy solar plexus chakra:

1. Too much self-focus
2. Thinking too much, distraction
3. Making, craving, grasping, clinging
4. "I know," holding on to ideas and convictions
5. Duality and opposites thinking, I and other, like and don't like
6. Past or future-oriented

The Traya practice has brought these into balance, but without regular meditation the mind energy "defaults" at the solar plexus chakra, and we cycle between these six forms of mind suffering. This chakra constructs a world to function in but we can become trapped in it. It is as if we build a house and never go out. I, my, me appears and we are constantly wanting, making, and constructing. Even when healthy, the solar plexus chakra has this tendency and we limit our spiritual options by our likes and don't likes—the teacher is not from Asia; the teacher is a man; the teacher is a woman; I don't like chanting in a different language, etc. All of these "manipurisms" keep us separate and in our own constructed world instead of experiencing the teachings and practices and seeing if they work for us. The solar plexus chakra makes judgments, whereas awareness allows things to be just the way they are. Daniella put it succinctly when she said (referring to meditation), "I can't get past thinking about it and actually do it; it never seems to be the right time or place." You can see the limiting manipurisms in this statement, "thinking" and "time," which inhibit being and doing. Thinking you already have the answers because of reading spiritual books is another manipurism—"I know."

When the higher chakras are "charged" by sustained meditation practice, then the "default" moves upwards, connects the crown chakra and the root chakra, and we experience freedom. The mind becomes calm, the ego quiets, and we let go of grasping and connect with the moment. The moment is the "holy grail" of Buddhism and yoga—the goal is to live more in our experiences, free of the solar plexus chakra's domination. Engagement with the higher chakras allows one to enter the spiritual dimension, expand consciousness, and gain new abilities. Energetically, when sitting in meditation we are downloading power, knowledge and stability from the universe through the crown chakra and uploading shakti, or grace, from the earth through the root chakra. Meditation is like charging the battery from two directions—earth and universe. Spirit comes from both mother earth and father sky as the Native Americans understood so clearly. If you are not plugged in, you cannot come fully alive. As you work with this practice, you come to understand that you really can trust the messages the Inner Teacher sends you, and you "stand in the lotus" and let go of grasping. The place where doing and being come together. To bloom fully we need spiritual food and nourishment. When you believe in yourself you are solid because then you believe in the higher self also.

Spiritual connection keeps us going with the Traya work, especially through any difficult parts of it. When we come out of the vicious circle of samskaric activity, we must now work on creating a virtuous circle fueled by spiritual connection. The Pathwork technique is an important tool for strengthening our connection to the spiritual path, showing us where we are slipping or lacking, and keeping us moving forward. The image that appears enables you to see if you are progressing. When I envisioned a path forward leading to spiritual growth, for example, I saw myself standing on the edge of a pier jutting out to a lake. Looking at this from the movement perspective (and that is the *most important information* in the Pathwork scene), unless I jump off the pier and start swimming I am not in a position to go forward (and I can't swim very fast nor far). Something is holding me back.

The next step in the Pathwork exercise is to then bring the attention to the body and ask, "Where in me is the energy that is slowing this path down?" I am drawn to the third eye chakra and the following comes up:

> … *You are too focused on the material world and denying the importance of the spiritual.*

I understand immediately why this is coming up. I have just come back from a visit to California to visit my daughter and granddaughter. We sometimes go for long walks near the water and admire the beautiful houses. I imagined living in one of those houses near them. The Manhattan neighborhood I live in has changed drastically over the years and has become a haven for the über wealthy. Our entire society seems to be racing to the top and many have a lot of money. It seems that materiality is the new religion and it can be difficult to stand aside and watch the race go by while barraged by ubiquitous messages that money and things bring happiness, while it seems that everyone else is buying in to it. More than 2,500 years ago, the prince and future Buddha left the palace and his lavish lifestyle, understanding that true happiness could not be found there, I realized that I too live in a palace not constructed of brick and mortar, but a society driven by consumerism and greed, and I need to step out of it as he did—at least in my mind.

The next time I did the Pathwork exercise (after I released society's attraction to the material world in the third eye chakra), I found myself in a rowboat on the lake, but I only had a stick and not a proper oar. This is how it works. The "path" changes as you release negative energy slowing it down—in this case blocking my spiritual progress. Being in a boat and having a stick is an improvement, but I am just drifting. So now I had to look and see what else was slowing me down. I take the Traya position and again ask what is slowing down the path and I am then led to the heart chakra:

> … *Growing up poor and always feeling unconsciously that everyone always had more than me.*

I have never resented others' wealth, but just felt that dynamic and now it was happening all over again.

Wealth indeed can be a separating energy—the rich separate themselves and the poor are separated from—both are extremes. It is the separating aspect that is the wound because the heart chakra's function is connection.

Truthfully, because of my meditation practice, I wasn't completely taken over by attachment to expensive homes, but my thoughts were sometimes stimulated by the lack dynamic from my childhood. I thought, "How will I be able to live near my daughter when I get older?" I released this lack energy in the heart chakra and check the path again.

Now I have an outboard motor but see myself pulling the cord and not hearing any whir. Now what? I am still not going anywhere but at least I have a boat. Back to Traya, where I am led to the crown chakra:

> …We have all been brainwashed to believe that "higher" spirituality requires moving to the mountain temples and living in seclusion. We are here to change the world and to do that we must live in it. To dig our roots in deep and bloom in the mud like the lotus. The lotus purifies the water it lives in and we must do the same.

Now I am acutely aware that I must examine how I live my daily life more closely and how my interactions with others and my example are so important. It is what happens off of the cushion that really matters. This is not the first time that I have heard this basic truth, but the difference is that now I own it. I check the path again and now I am in a speedboat flying across the water. The movement tells me that I am now on track but I must check in often as things can change and something different may distract me from my focus on spiritual growth.

Watching the Mind

Watching our minds is another tool. We may first practice Traya in order to eliminate gross afflictions and may not notice the more subtle ones. As we purify the mind, we become aware of more subtle forms of negativity that on the surface do not appear to be harming us. These often appear in our yoga class or on meditation retreats.

The most egregious of these for me was after I entered a spiritual yoga class at Integral Yoga and having just left Zen practice.

Everyone rolls out their mats—about twelve people—and the teacher asks us to first sit cross-legged for some preliminary chanting. It is a hot spring day and the ceiling fans are on and the breeze feels good. The teacher asks if everyone is comfortable with the ceiling fans on, and a woman across and to the left says, "No, I am cold—turn off the fans."

No one objected so the teacher turned off the fans. I am thinking, "That woman is a gym yoga type—she even looks like a gym yoga type and doesn't care if the rest of us are hot or not." The teacher started the chanting and I heard a cell phone go off and it sounded like it came from the "gym yoga" woman's direction. She didn't answer. Next I heard *ting, ting*—the noise that lets you know that there is a voicemail message to pick up. "Oh no," I thought, "we are going to have to hear this throughout the entire class—that is too much and the gym yoga woman is not moving to turn off her cell phone—how inconsiderate. I went up to the teacher and said, "Will you please ask whoever has their cell phone beeping to turn it off?" And he made this announcement to the class.

However, we are all sitting in opposite rows and no one moved. I look at the gym yoga woman and she doesn't move. I look up and down the rows and everyone is just sitting. I hear "ting" again and realize, "Oh no!" and go over to my bag to take out my cell phone and turn it off! I had just come from meditation practice and "I, my, me" was front and center—big time. But the difference is that I saw it clearly (of course, I was hit over the head with it) and I saw that this "gym" yoga woman is a great teacher. I didn't think to do Traya with this but vowed to be aware of my tendency to judge and jump to conclusions about people.

Meditation retreats too have a way of bringing a lot of this to our attention. A friend told me of her "yellow pants" story. She was away at a long retreat and had brought along her favorite yellow pants that were nice and loose and comfortable to sit in. There was a shared laundry facility and often people's clean things would get taken out of the dryer and mixed up in a large basket. She went to get ready for practice one day and couldn't find her yellow pants. When she arrived in the meditation room, she saw that the woman bowing in front of her was wearing her yellow pants. She couldn't focus on the practice for the entire session, thinking, how could this woman do this? It was a silent retreat so she was at odds of what to do about it.

My friend went and looked in the laundry basket, but her pants weren't there. "They have to be mine," she thought. "How many people have yellow pants? And I can't find mine." The retreat lasted the entire weekend and the woman wore the yellow pants the entire time. My friend was so agitated she snuck out of the retreat and called a friend asking what she should do. The friend wisely advised her not to do anything until the end of the retreat and to try to let it go in the meantime. She had great difficulty meditating and felt that the retreat was ruined for her. She was going over in her mind what she would say to the woman and was also anticipating her reaction. After the last practice period on the last day, she was in her room packing and, lo and behold, she found her yellow pants. She had spent so much time constructing her version that she actually thought that the woman had somehow snuck the pants back into her bag when she wasn't around. She rushed out to confront the woman and saw her wearing the yellow pants.

Even teachers as wise and experienced as Pema Chödrön can fall into this trap and she relates a similar story in her book *Start Where You Are*. She had been leading a retreat. During a break, she went to the kitchen and was angered to see dirty dishes in the sink. She thought of a likely suspect. "Who did she think was going to wash these dishes, her mother?" Then she picked up a dirty dish and saw her own name, Pema, on it—and on the cup and knife!

Several years after my yoga cell phone incident, I was in a hot yoga class that was very crowded with men on both sides of me. I became aware of a sweat odor and said to myself, "I don't understand why men think they can come to class without wearing deodorant—they just don't care about the people around them." Then we were doing a pose that required the arms to be up and I realized the smell was coming from me! I forgot to put on deodorant before I went out! "I did it again," I realized. I thought that my awareness from the cell phone incident was going to prevent this and it didn't. This time I did Traya with it and was led to the solar plexus chakra:

> ...*People around me often spoke badly of other people.*
> ...*My father was a big man and when he sneezed the whole house would shake and it felt like an ambush.*

This time I was able to release the energy that drives this mindset. This shows that even beyond symptoms, we must keep purifying the mind.

One of my Zen teachers used the analogy of a potato peeling machine to describe this phenomena. It is like putting the potatoes in the machine and turning it on and the potatoes fly around and are peeled by rubbing up against each other. Retreat participants rub up against each other and this allows us to see what we are holding in our minds more clearly. How can we explain the similarity in the types of responses to others after meditation in all three of the above stories? We can see our solar plexus chakra's tendency to separate "I" and "other" and to judge, construct stories, and jump to conclusions. The solar plexus chakra likes to dominate our mind and to be in control, and when we are working hard in meditation to escape its clutches, it tries to pull us back in and we may slip temporarily. A good antidote (besides doing more Traya to heal this reactivity and judgementalism in the solar plexus chakra) is to keep the attention at the pelvic chakra beyond the influence of the solar plexus—breathe in and out and/or repeat its seed sound, vam.

We can also use Traya to deepen our meditation practice. On a meditation retreat, I became acutely aware of watching the clock, thinking about the food that was to come later and sleeping as long as I wanted the next day. I realized that I tend to live in the future, when I get off of work I can do this, I will have this for dinner, etc. Planning is OK but when these thoughts come up frequently, there is something else going on and I knew that this went on in my mind a lot of the time. I followed this to mukta, the letting go chakra, and learned:

> …*I was holding on to the future as a way of escaping an unpleasant present. When I was a kid, life was unpleasant and I held on to the future in anticipation of escaping it.*

Although my present was no longer unpleasant, I couldn't relax into it because of the "holding energy" in the letting go chakra taking me out. The letting go chakra is associated with manipura, the solar plexus chakra—the time creator, so it used time as a mechanism to do this. When I let this energy go, the thoughts ceased and I relaxed into my experience of the retreat. As with any Traya healing, the result held and I no longer live life in constant anticipation of the next experience and am more able to live in the moment.

We can meditate and try to detach from these types of things or we can remove them so that they don't come up at all and pull us off track. I was meditating to stay in the moment and I was continually being pulled into the future. In Zen we meditate so that we don't bite the hook, but if the hook isn't there then our ability to be present in meditation and in our lives deepens.

So purification of the mind requires awareness of all types of negativity, from gross symptoms such as fear to negative thoughts of all types, whether or not they feel hurtful to ourselves.

When we shift our focus from the external to internal, we balance. It is a seeming paradox that when we put emphasis on the internal we are actually more engaged in the world—and happily so, for we have developed beneficial qualities such as kindness, compassion, equanimity, mindfulness, courage, hopefulness, clarity, and determination that make living a joyful experience. And not just for us. Similar to how our Traya practice has been fruitful, these new qualities and our emphasis on continued spiritual growth bear fruit in the outside world—we become clearer as to how we can help.

Like meditation and yoga, Traya is a practice that has benefits that may seem incomprehensible, but if we are wise, we hold them close. One doesn't have to become a Buddhist or embrace all of yoga philosophy—it is the meditation and yoga *practice* that connects us to spiritual energy. Practicing meditation and yoga with others has a special benefit as we pick up spiritual energy from the practice, the place of practice, and from other practitioners. Like meditation and yoga, you can only understand Traya with experience. We enter the stage of transformation when we deepen our meditation and yoga practice, watch our minds, and focus on our spiritual path. What a privilege it is to have the tools to deal with past karma!

While on this journey, we will be continuously changing and growing. It is crucial to remember that spiritual growth, blooming our spiritual lotus, and doing our true work involves staying in the moment. So we have the connection to the moment and a future goal at the same time. This may appear paradoxical. Like the root chakra, the spiritual path involves action and movement and, at the same time, staying in the moment. Connecting with everyday experience right now, moment by moment, we can use that experience to feed our blooming Lotus of Full Potential.

Part 2
UNDERSTANDING AND WORKING WITH EACH OF THE CHAKRAS USING TRAYA

Each of the following seven chapters is devoted to one of the primary chakras and its associated secondary chakra(s). Together these chapters form a map guiding us on a journey through the inner landscape of the mind, with many twists and turns and mysteries revealed.

If you are familiar with the chakras from prior reading or study, you will not be surprised to see, for example, that the throat chakra has to do with communication and the root chakra with safety and security. I have discovered additional attributes of the primary chakras along with the secondary chakras and their functions through Traya exploration both with myself and others.

This discovery process was the result of many years of careful listening and attention to detail, quite like old time mapmaking before satellites and GPS, where charting a region required rigorous and time-consuming exploration and documentation with no shortcuts. Only this time we were traveling through the deep space of the mind. As similar material appeared related to a specific chakra, I was able to expand the list. For example, when different people surfaced memories related to injustice when working with the solar plexus chakra, I realized that one of its attributes is a sense of justice. I also discovered that the primary chakras each have one function and several attributes and the secondaries have just the one function without attributes.

At the beginning of each chapter, I note the chakra function, a comprehensive list of its attributes, and the common issues that result from negative samskaras. I also include, for illustrative purposes, an example of an attribute paradox for that chakra. An attribute paradox occurs when an attribute of a chakra is samskaric and contradicts the chakras function. For example, the jolly man or woman who uses humor to entertain others in order to be liked—the pelvic chakra function is associated with personal power in relationships, and this misuse of its attribute of humor is in contradiction to personal power.

Some of the material may be controversial, especially in the crown chakra, in relation to religion, culture, and society. It is important to understand the types of experiences that cause injuries to the mind so that we can know why we have the wounds that we do and prevent wounding other people.

Change is always happening, whether or not an issue is completely resolved. As previously noted, when one chakra is significantly out of balance there will be issues in other chakras as well. Think of tuning a piano; for it to be tuned properly, more than one string needs to be adjusted. There are tipping points throughout the process when enough samskaras related to a particular issue are healed and there is a sudden and dramatic positive change in the mind. Thus, change is both gradual and sudden. One is obvious and one is not so obvious; therefore, I do not mention change with every example. Chapter 5 provides a general outline of the types of changes that can be expected when addressing a dominant pain body.

How to Approach This Work

If you have a substantial pain body, I recommend that the lower chakras be cleansed of samskaras first so that there is a foundation established to allow the higher chakras to bloom. I always prefer starting with the solar plexus chakra as its separating and intellectualizing tendency will be reduced. This helps with work on the spiritual path and with the Traya process. It is also the easiest chakra for beginners to work with as we are all very comfortable and familiar with the solar plexus chakra's "in our head" energy. This is the order (top down) that I suggest:

- The solar plexus chakra (manipura)
- The pelvic chakra (svadhisthana)
- The throat chakra (vishuddha)
- The root chakra (muladhara)
- The heart chakra (anahata)
- The third eye chakra (ajna)
- The crown chakra (sahasrara)

The solar plexus chakra, the pelvic chakra, and the throat chakra, when samskaric, cause many unpleasant thoughts and feelings. The root chakra goes next because one should be fully grounded with a strong foundation before the higher chakras (heart, throat, third eye, and crown) are strengthened.

Of course, if you review the primary chakra list in chapter 2 and realize that you are significantly out of balance in one area, for example, your doing energy is very weak and you struggle to get yourself moving—work in that area until you are functioning better—in this case the root chakra. I still would recommend alternating one day the solar plexus chakra and then the next day the identified problem chakra. For many of us, it is essential that the solar plexus chakra is brought into balance, as early in the process as possible. When the solar plexus chakra is balanced we are able to engage more fully with every aspect of life, including this process, as we are less likely to be thwarted by excessive thinking, distractions, and judgments.

If your pain body is not substantial, work in areas you are drawn to or where you are led by your Inner Teacher. Sometimes you may even be led to work on a higher chakra or to focus on one of the secondary chakras; trust yourself. The secondary chakras are small but powerful and can provide much relief from negativity in the mind. Work on these whenever you are led to them.

Goals are good, but in the beginning try to work with negative thoughts or feelings and, then later in the process, patterns of behavior.

It is a good idea to keep a notebook and record every change that you notice as you notice them. If you are working with an issue such as fear, draw a line with numbers along the line ranging from 0 to 10. Rate your average fear level in the beginning on that line with 10 being the severest and 0 representing no fear at all. Check in from time to time and think of how fearful you have been feeling in the past week in general. Record each change until the fear decreases to 0. Of course this will take time if you fall high on the fear range, and it is important to stay cognizant of progress because as the mind shifts we can forget what it was like before and become frustrated as the focus turns to other issues. Sara put this well: "I was driving in my car and another car came out of nowhere, and I felt a panicked feeling. Later I realized that I used to feel like this all of the time. I was walking around with an underlying constant fear that would bubble up into panic at times. After doing the Traya work, it is hard for me to even remember what that was like as I am not like that now."

There are exercises included to aid you in your beginning work with both the primary and secondary chakras discussed in each chapter. These exercises together include all of the various techniques for locating samskaras that were outlined in chapter 3 on the Traya process so that you can get some experience with all of them. Feel free, however, to stick with the basic technique. Remember that this is a simple process. The memory comes up and the energy goes out—that is basically it. I have made every effort not to complicate things. It is only the various methods you can use to locate samskaras in the chakras that can change—the other Traya steps are always the same.

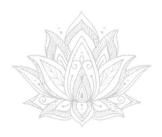

Chapter 6

THE ROOT CHAKRA (MULADHARA)
AND THE IMAGINATION CHAKRA (ATILOKA)

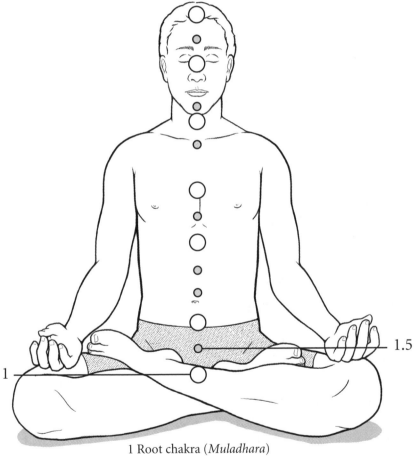

1 Root chakra (*Muladhara*)
1.5 Imagination chakra (*Atiloka*)

Figure 6: First Chakra

Muladhara, the Root Chakra

- **Function:** safety and security in physical environment
- **Attributes:** doing, embodiment, grounding, action, movement, accomplishment, standing up for oneself, moment connection, manifestation, kundalini shakti
- **Attribute paradox:** "I can't accomplish what I want because I am doing too much."
- **Common issues in muladhara:** lack of grounding, difficulty standing up for oneself, procrastination, overcoming obstacles, staying in the moment

The root chakra connects us to the physical world, including our own body. We need to take action to make sure that our needs are met so we can survive in the physical environment. However, this doing energy must be balanced, otherwise, as in the attribute paradox from earlier, it will instead get in the way of accomplishment.

Physical Safety and Security, "Bodyfullness," Grounding

When you don't feel safe you can't ground completely because you need to be able to move quickly. Grounding requires feeling safe enough to make a commitment to the moment as well as putting your energy into it.

It is through this chakra that we connect to the earth, to the material world, to our surroundings and to our bodies. At birth and shortly thereafter, children sense whether or not they are in a safe place with their needs being met. If they feel that security, they become fully embodied. As the child grows and further experiences the environment, that sense of safety and security strengthens or weakens. Disharmony or danger in the outside environment or in the home environment causes the body and earth connection to weaken.

An example of experiences that will damage this energy is that of Sara, who was adopted when she was an infant and was also teased in school. She has a good job yet complains of having an "undercurrent of insecurity" in her life. We surfaced the following unconscious material at the root chakra:

> *...I don't know what grounded is. I can't trust or count on anything. I always have to perform.*
> *...I had a recurring nightmare of my mom putting me back on the bus to send me back—I WAS UPROOTED.*
> *...I always feel, you are not welcome here, always afraid I will wear out my welcome.*

She was literally uprooted from her birth mother and home, damaging this energy and producing an abiding sense of insecurity instead of security.

The earth has hard and soft aspects, rocks and grass. In the body this is also true as there are both the hard skeletal structure and soft tissues. In the Traya work with Jim, it came to him that he didn't have any structure growing up. His parents were busy and would let him do whatever he wanted. After he released that energy he said, "I feel a palpable shift in connection to my body, really quite wonderful. I could feel my separation from my body and then it disappeared as my body and mind integrated. A very wonderful feeling." Then he said, "I also didn't receive much soft touch either." So we processed that and he then felt even more embodied and grounded.

Doing Energy

Sheila complains about procrastinating around tasks at home. She will, at times, get a short burst of energy and clean the whole house but will then again revert to lying around for days at a time. She feels out of balance and powerless to change it. Traya exploration revealed the following samskara contributing to this imbalance:

> *...My mother was like the energizer bunny—working a full-time job and then coming home and cooking and cleaning and caring for three kids. She would literally collapse on the couch after we were all taken care of. My father sat and watched TV and never lifted a finger to help.*

Sheila's "doing energy" is out of balance because doing energy was out of balance in her home growing up, and she picked up that unbalanced energy. After Traya work, her doing and resting energy came into balance and she stopped procrastinating.

When we think about issues with getting things done, we often conjure images of the couch potato–type rather than the workaholic type, because constantly working hard is highly valued in our society. In fact both the couch potato and the workaholic are out of balance in that both are missing out on important parts of life—the couch potato, the joys and gains of productivity; and the workaholic, the joys and benefits of rest, relationships, and recreation.

A word in defense of the unproductive and the couch potatoes of this world: I don't believe that there is such a thing as a lazy person—only a person with impacted "doing energy." If the root chakra is healthy, there is *always* action and productivity. Not only are we doing and accomplishing, but we are doing what we really *need* to do.

Standing Up for Oneself

To be firmly grounded and rooted is to be like a strong tree with deep roots that can't be pushed over. People with weak root chakras have difficulty standing up for themselves with others. This energy helps one to stand up for oneself in the moment rather than having a delayed reaction. Lisa reported that she noticed that when someone was rude by slamming a store door in her face as she was coming through with packages, it didn't fully register with her until she was on the street waiting for the bus, and then she reacted with annoyance. The rude person was long gone. The French have a term for this—*l'esprit de l'escalier*—which refers to thinking of a retort while on the stairs having already left the party.

Gloria, the victim of severe physical bullying as a young child, after healing this chakra stated, "I feel more rooted, grounded, and sure of myself. So different I can't believe it." She then started standing up for herself at work, where she had been feeling positively overwhelmed and often complained about it. She wrote a proposal for the redistribution of the work, including more delegation, and presented it to her supervisor, who readily accepted it.

Overcoming Obstacles and Manifestation

Ganesh is the Hindu deity that is associated with this chakra. He is known as the "Remover of Obstacles." When this energy is strong, obstacles on one's path are easily avoided or overcome. The root chakra is one of the three Manifestation Chakras—the crown and heart chakras are the other two. The root chakra connects to the earth energy that is always manifesting new life. This energy is key because if our roots are not strong, earth energy cannot flow into our subtle body and the things that we are trying to manifest will lack energy and be stunted. The root chakra keeps things moving; earth energy is constantly in motion, always growing and changing and creating—slowly, like the movement of the elephant, but unstoppable.

Connection to Moment

When this energy is strong, we are connected to the moment, less spacey, and more detail-oriented. Everything happens in the moment, and if we are not connected to it, we miss out.

Kundalini Shakti

Kundalini spiritual energy lies dormant in this chakra until it is awakened by spiritual practices such as yoga and meditation. You can think of kundalini as a coiled snake that, when awakened, rises up the sushumna nadi and activates the crown chakra. See chapter 4 for further discussion of kundalini.

Imagination Chakra (Atiloka)

- **Location:** a few inches above the pubic bone between the root chakra (muladhara) and the pelvic chakra (svadhisthana)
- **Function:** imagination

This secondary chakra lifts the mind above the mundane material world consciousness. It brings people, magic, and fun into life. In this chakra, the imagination springs forth and we use the creative energy of the pelvic chakra to perceive or imagine magical beings or special energies that inhabit the physical world (root chakra) with us. Stories of fairies and nature spirits "lighten up" and add color to the everyday world of basic survival. Every culture has this phenomenon and/or perceives a subtle essence in the natural surroundings. Trees, rocks, and rivers are imbued with spirit and are seen as more than just the physical elements they contain. In the imagination chakra, a relationship to the enchanted realm becomes part of human consciousness.

The pelvic chakra has to do with relationships and the imagination chakra provides the "lift and impetus" to get out into the world and socialize rather than just focus on doing tasks related to home and survival.

Sheila complains that her life doesn't have any spark. She comes home from work and focuses on accomplishing things around the house and claims she is too busy to socialize. She cannot understand how others manage a social life in this "demanding world we live in." In exploring the imagination chakra she came upon the following:

…Growing up we were always focused on survival issues as we were always on the brink. I remember my socks didn't match and at one point I had cardboard in my shoes. I tried to forget it when I was with my friends but it was hard as there seemed to always be an issue about money. My parents worked hard but at low-paying jobs and they never had time to socialize at all.

It is clear that this material is appropriate for the imagination chakra because it is related to both the root chakra (survival) below and the pelvic chakra (social) above. This is not the only energy contributing to Sheila's difficulty socializing, of course, but it is an important piece of the puzzle and she did notice more of an interest in socializing after our session.

When you are focused on survival, it is difficult to enjoy life. The imagination chakra moves us to pursue relief from the drudgery of the work-a-day world and encourages us to dance through life. To take a creative approach rather than stay stuck in routine and habit. If thinking about nature spirits is too "out there" for you, think about how you feel when you get lost in a good book or movie. These are modern ways to escape from our daily duties and chores. And you then have good conversation material for use with others you encounter in the social realm of the pelvic chakra. After all, no one likes to talk about work at cocktail parties!

••• EXERCISE: TRAYA PRACTICE AT THE ••• ROOT CHAKRA (MULADHARA)

Grounding

It is good to ground oneself in the body at the beginning and end of each Traya session. Do this by sitting up straight and focusing on the soles of your feet. Imagine breathing in and out from there.

Basic Technique

We will use the basic technique in which we focus on a chakra and ask, "What memories are here?"

Step 1: Focus—Keep your attention at the pubic bone and breathe in and out gently.

Step 2: Surface—Adopt the letting stance and ask, "What memories are here?"

Step 3: Release—Note the memory and start to let negative energy go out by visualizing it coming out of the chakra. Then either go back to step 2 and surface another memory and then repeat step 3 or proceed to step 4. Note that you do not have to let all of the energy from the previous memory go out before you surface the next one. You are continuously adding to the outflow of negative energy memory by memory—like adding links to a chain. After you are finished surfacing memories for this session, let all the negative energy go out and wait until the outflow stops.

Step 4: Replace and Imprint—Visualize positive energy coming in (rays from the sun) and taking up the space that was taken up by the negative energy that went out. Ask, "What is this positive energy bringing in with it?" Note the words that appear in your mind.

Step 5: Scene from Nature (Optional)—Breathe in and out while focusing attention on the root chakra and let a scene from nature appear in your mind. Note if the earth energy element is strong. (See pages 34–35 for scene from nature guide.)

Finish by grounding again.

••• EXERCISE: TRAYA PRACTICE AT THE ••• IMAGINATION CHAKRA (ATILOKA)

The basic technique was used in the earlier root chakra exercise. Let's use the manifestation technique (page 47) for locating samskaras in a chakra this time. This technique is based on the Traya inside/outside rule—to find what is inside a chakra, we only need to look outside and vice versa. Perhaps you are aware that you tend to not like to participate in games or play sports. Or you are one of those people who only like to read history and not light-hearted or fantastical narratives. You would review the chart in chapter 2 and see where these issues might be located and you trace them to the imagination chakra. Next is to continue with the Traya practice. You ground by breathing in and out of the soles of your feet.

Step 1: Focus—Keep your attention a few inches above the pubic bone and breathe in and out gently.

Step 2: Surface—Adopt the letting stance and ask, "What memories are here?"

Step 3: Release—Note the memory and start to let negative energy go out by visualizing it coming out of the chakra. Then either go back to step 2 and surface another memory and then repeat step 3, or continue to step 4. Keep surfacing memories and adding to the chain of negative energy going out.

Step 4: Replace and Imprint—Visualize positive energy coming in (rays from the sun) and taking up the space that was taken up by the negative energy that went out. Ask, "What is this positive energy bringing in with it?" Note the words that appear in your mind.

Ground. (There is no scene from nature step with the secondary chakras.)

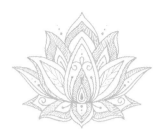

Chapter 7

THE PELVIC CHAKRA (SVADHISTHANA) AND THE FEARLESS CHAKRA (ABHAYA)

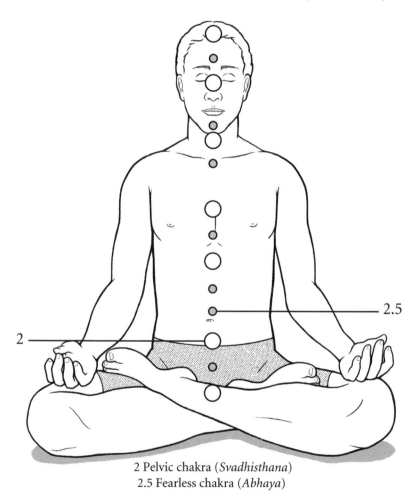

2 Pelvic chakra (*Svadhisthana*)
2.5 Fearless chakra (*Abhaya*)

Figure 7: Second Chakra

Svadhisthana, the Pelvic Chakra

- **Function:** personal power in relationships
- **Attributes:** centeredness, poise, dignity, charisma, sexual and emotional energy, buoyancy, self-possession, boundaries, creativity, humor
- **Attribute paradox:** "I make them laugh so they will like me."
- **Common issues in svadhisthana:** caring too much what others think, poor boundaries, lack of access to anger, boredom

We are relational beings. We group together for fun and for protection as there is strength in numbers. We have different kinds of relationships—spousal, relatives, neighbors, friends, teachers, students, coworkers, and members of every group or organization that we associate with. How we find our place in these groups without losing ourselves is the business of the pelvic chakra—the social center where we orient ourselves in society.

Known in Taoism, Buddhism, and martial arts as the *dantian* (in Chinese, meaning "energy garden" or "elixir field"), *tanjon* (in Korean), and *hara* (in Japanese), it is the seat of the *chi* or *qi* (prana) in the subtle body. It is our center of physical gravity. Martial arts practitioners and meditators are advised to keep their attention here to quiet, stabilize, and focus the mind—thus, the pejorative "navel-gazer."

Downward-flowing earth prana is governed by the root chakra, while in this pelvic center the energy flow is interpersonal. Rivers and oceans provide natural boundaries in the physical world and personal boundaries are an attribute here. A flowing river produces power— mechanical and electrical in the natural world and personal in this energy field. It is the "generator" of the energy system and supplies vigor for our lives.

When you think about the pelvic chakra, think, "How do I feel about myself in relation to others? Do I care too much about what others think?" Here we relate to society, and public opinion is a force that holds society together.

Emotions, Boundaries, and Personal Power

This chakra provides the energy for stabilizing the emotions. How anger is handled is significant here. Positive anger—anger that is not driven by samskaras—can be an energetic mechanism for staking out boundaries and defending one's dignity. "My feelings are just as important as yours, and I can take up emotional space in the world."

Often people feel caught in a polarity between appeasement and rage, i.e., "I will take the high road because if I get angry, either I will explode and ruin everything or the other person will." There is no middle place—no balance—no healthy anger. This is the pelvic chakra out of balance. When there is bad behavior on the part of someone else, instead of anger there is appeasement. One starts to question oneself. "Was I disrespected or not? Did they really mean what they said? Do I have a right to feel this way? Maybe they didn't really mean it? Well they are going through a bad time, I don't want to make it worse by getting angry at them?" The sense of ownership of one's feelings is impeded and one is out of touch with one's own personal power—that is, one attaches more importance to others' thoughts and feelings than one's own.

Stefano was hampered in his relationship because he was frequently putting his girlfriend's needs ahead of his. She was often demanding and critical of him. Traya exploration revealed that at age eleven his parents had an acrimonious divorce and they are still at odds fifteen years later. As a teenager he often acted as the go-between to obtain money or "settle" things. By using Stefano in this manner, his parents were disregarding his intense but hidden feelings and sending the message "Our feelings are more important than yours." They were getting to express their anger at each other and in doing that indirectly through him were sending him the message "Your feelings don't count." The samskaras produced by this behavior suppressed his ability to connect with his anger and his personal power was dampened. After she broke up with him, during Traya work he stated:

… You know, there were several things about this girl that I sensed in the beginning. Several ways that she insulted me but that I let slide. If I had paid more attention, I would have been out of there before it even got going.

He was aware of her behavior but *excused* it. If he had personal power, he would have experienced his anger and asked himself, "Do I want to be around someone who disrespects me," because anger would have let him know that he was being disrespected. Instead he was focused on what he was doing to provoke her.

How do we relate to others and still maintain our personal boundaries? Boundaries define relationships—you get your needs met but not at the expense of mine and vice versa. Both physical and emotional space is important in this chakra and having "one's own" space is key to a healthy svadhisthana, which literally means "one's own." A few examples of samskaric experiences related to physical and emotional space that disrupt this energy:

Raina: *…I was never able to make my room my own—nothing was mine—Mother always decorated—there was no freedom to do anything like that.*

Gloria: *…My father is in his head—like his emotions are missing—He told my mother when she was crying in the movies, "Don't make an exhibit of yourself."*

Frequent arguing and angry outbursts also are boundary violations because they take up the emotional space in the home and there is no room for the other family members' emotions. The last memory is also related to taking up emotional space. The message is "emotions are not allowed." There is no room for them. The father was disconnected from his own emotions and this also sends a message that emotions are not safe or welcome. When she cried, she was told to "put a lid on it." As a result Gloria was unable to access her anger. She would have the idea of anger but not the feeling. The ability to feel anger is an important pelvic chakra function. Anger is a powerful emotion that enables the defense of boundaries. Without it, Gloria is unable to defend her boundaries.

"All of my life I have been treated as though my feelings don't matter," she said.

When she released enough samskaras from the pelvic chakra, she stated that she felt fully alive and able to take up space for the first time. She expanded her creative boundaries by successfully networking with more and more people related to a personal project important to her.

Poor boundaries will sometimes manifest in the tendency to violate other people's space or to reveal too much personal information before one has gotten to know another.

Boundary issues are particularly difficult for women as in many societies it is considered de rigueur to violate a woman's personal boundaries with street comments, unwanted sexual attention, sexual jokes and innuendo, and even overt touching or grabbing. Almost every woman that I have ever worked with, including myself, had to heal samskaras related to some of these types of experiences to reclaim their personal power and find boundary balance in relationships.

Focus on the Other

Every experience has an impact and the following demonstrates how there doesn't have to be "trauma" to produce samskaras. This experience is dissonant to the function of the chakra and shifts the focus from self to the other.

Karen is a young woman from the Midwest who is married and attending journalism graduate school in New York. There are difficulties in her marriage related to her husband's lack of access to his emotions and his desire to be taken care of. In beginning to work on relationship issues here at the pelvic chakra, the following memory came up:

...I am five years old at a country picnic with a large group of family and friends. When we are leaving, I can't find my new sweater. In the car going home I am crying and my mother says

that she knows who took it but doesn't want to embarrass them or make a scene.

Her mother didn't stand up for her and, instead, put the stealing person's needs ahead of Karen's. The message here is fourfold: (1) appease others, (2) your needs are not as important as other people's, (3) avoid conflict at all costs, and (4) suppress your anger.

This brings up an important point—samskaras are deposited not only from situations such as the earlier discussed but from "picking them up" from parents with impaired power energy. We pick up samskaras from our environment just as we do biological viruses. Powerlessness means that outside forces are in charge. We can also give our power away to instruments of society such as organizations, money, or substances.

Sara was talking about how she thinks about relationships with the emphasis on what she will lose or give up if she gets in a relationship. "I have never had the initiative to date and look out for my needs—always wanting to meet theirs." Traya revealed:

> *…All my favorite music up to the day I was divorced was based on what the guy I was in a relationship with liked. Who do you want me to be? I was like a collage of what I thought other people wanted.*
> *…Age sixteen, my boyfriend shoved me—warning signs that I ignored.*
> *…Nothing in me was willing to honor what I needed.*

Charles put it well: "I put others' needs first and expect that they will eventually do the same for me, but that never happens." It never will because, in putting others' needs first there is the implicit communication that one's own needs are unimportant.

Sexual Energy

Sex is something we do with another person, whether in person or in the head. "It takes two to tango," so to speak. Sexual energy can be misdirected, suppressed, or otherwise made dysfunctional by samskaras in the pelvic chakra.

An extreme example is people who sell their bodies for money. They are typically able to do so because their personal boundaries have already been compromised, often by sexual abuse, or they are disconnected in other essential ways from themselves. The psyche is wholesome and doesn't abide any unwholesome activities, so more and more samskaras are deposited by this activity.

Sometimes sexual energy can be entangled with other samskaras, an unavailable parent, for example—and one will feel an extreme sexual attraction toward unavailable people. Be careful with unusually strong sexual attractions; they may be a red flag.

Buoyancy
When healthy, the pelvic chakra provides an upbeat type of energy. When unhealthy, one can feel bored and have difficulty becoming excited about projects or life. Boredom can also be an issue in the solar plexus chakra, but that is the boredom that comes from the inability to engage fully due to distancing energy. In the pelvic chakra, it lingers from childhood experiences of boredom. Jim states:

> *…I was beaten down by boredom. My friends and I acted out constantly out of sheer boredom.*

Fearless Chakra (Abhaya)

• **Location:** one inch above navel
• **Function:** unafraid of others' power

Abhaya lies between the pelvic chakra (relations with other people) and the solar plexus chakra (can produce fear), so abhaya governs fear (or not) of other people's influence and power.

Aimee is a young aspiring actress originally from France. Aimee wanted to feel more embodied and centered while performing in her acting classes. When she goes on stage, she is more concerned with pleasing the teacher rather than focusing on the work. We found that her fearless chakra was samskaric because of the excessive power imbalance in her relationship to her parents. Some of the memories and insights that came up in her Traya work at this chakra related to her parents but especially her mother:

> ...*I had no rights to my feelings. I should just be grateful and thankful.*
> ...*Mother was always comparing me to others negatively.*
> ...*I am afraid of not living up to others' expectations. Mom was good at academics and I failed miserably.*

As we released these and other related samskaras, she began to feel more sure of herself, connected to her center and present in the moment. Her acting improved because she said, "I am more me."

••• EXERCISE: TRAYA PRACTICE AT THE ••• PELVIC CHAKRA (SVADHISTHANA)

Grounding
Ground by sitting up straight, focusing on the soles of your feet, and breathing in and out of the tertiary chakras in the feet.

Follow the Body Technique
With this technique, you let the deep mind direct you to a location to work on. There are two ways to do this. After grounding, you can just focus on the body and ask, "Where in me is there any energy that needs to move?" Or you can either think of an issue, let's say feeling uncomfortable in groups, for example. And you ask, "Where in me is the energy related to this?" Using either technique you are led to the pelvic chakra because you feel a sensation there. You then continue with the Traya steps.

> **Step 1: Focus**—Keep your attention one inch below the navel and breathe in and out gently.
> **Step 2: Surface**—Adopt the letting stance and ask, "What memories are here?"

Step 3: Release—Note the memory and start to let negative energy go out by visualizing it coming out of the chakra. Then either go back to step 2 and surface another memory and then repeat step 3 or proceed to step 4. Note that you do not have to let all the energy from the previous memory go out before you surface the next one. You are continuously adding to the outflow of negative energy memory by memory—like adding links to a chain. After you are finished surfacing memories for this session, let all of the negative energy go out and wait until the outflow stops.

Step 4: Replace and Imprint—Visualize positive energy coming in (rays from the sun) and taking up the space that was taken up by the negative energy that went out. Ask, "What is this positive energy bringing in with it?" Note the words that appear in your mind.

Step 5: Scene from Nature (Optional)—Breathe in and out while focusing attention on the pelvic chakra and let a scene from nature appear in your mind. Note if the water element is strong. (See chapter 2 list of chakra elements.) Finish by grounding again.

••• EXERCISE: TRAYA PRACTICE AT THE ••• FEARLESS CHAKRA (ABHAYA)

You use the follow the body technique we just reviewed and you are led to abhaya about one inch above the navel. Next is to continue with the Traya practice. You ground by breathing in and out of the soles of your feet.

Step 1: Focus—Keep your attention on abhaya one inch above the navel and breathe in and out gently.

Step 2: Surface—Adopt the letting stance and ask, "What memories are here?"

Step 3: Release—Note the memory and start to let negative energy go out by visualizing it coming out of the chakra. Then either go back to step 2 and surface another memory and then repeat step 3 or proceed to step 4. Keep surfacing memories and adding to the chain of negative energy going out.

Step 4: Replace and Imprint—Visualize positive energy coming in (rays from the sun) and taking up the space that was taken up by the negative energy that went out. Ask, "What is this positive energy bringing in with it?" Note the words that appear in your mind.

Ground again. There is no scene from nature step, as this is a secondary chakra.

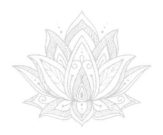

Chapter 8

THE SOLAR PLEXUS CHAKRA (MANIPURA) AND THE RELEASE CHAKRA (MUKTA)

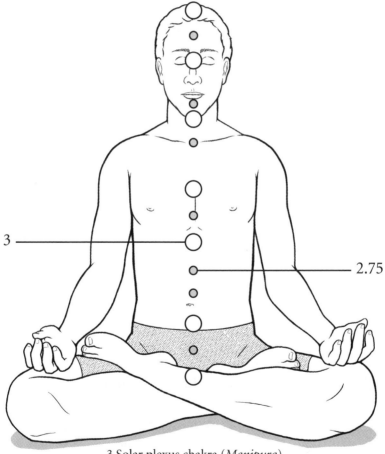

3 Solar plexus chakra (*Manipura*)
2.75 Release chakra (*Mukta*)

Figure 8: Third Chakra

Manipura, the Solar Plexus Chakra

- **Function:** I-consciousness
- **Attributes:** ego, intellect, structure, logic, reasoning, reality testing, will, drive, determination, duality, direction, orientation in
time and place, courage, clarity, ease, flexibility, decision-making,
problem-solving, calm, engagement, justice, fairness, balance, self-
control, open mind, vitality, going with the flow, ability to focus
- **Attribute paradox:** "My thoughts define me."
- **Common issues in manipura:** too much thinking, fear, worry,
sense of isolation, disengaged, distracted

The solar plexus chakra governs the thinking faculty and the ego,
enabling logical, analytic, and rational thinking as well as the ability
to plan. Some authors locate it at or near the navel and others place it
at the solar plexus. I have found it to be definitely at the diaphragm in
front of the solar plexus. When we locate the thinking process in our
bodies, we often point to our brains, but the mechanism that supports
and balances the thinking faculty is actually located in manipura at
the solar plexus. The ancient Greeks agree, and our language also supports this perspective:

> The Greek in Homeric times located his thinking a bit below
> the heart, in the diaphragm. Another word for diaphragm is
> *phren*, the Greek word for mind; and the same root is in the
> name of the mental disease schizo*phren*ia, which means a split-
> ting of the mind. So in the Homeric days, the physical localiza-
> tion of the mind was in the region of the diaphragm.[10]

The solar plexus chakra is analogous with what we have come
to think of as the "left brain"—the part of the mind that imposes a
structure on our world, creating the subject/object distance and attempting to understand the world through the intellect by labeling
and categorizing. For example, the tendency of humans to look at the

---

10. Sonu Shamdasani, *The Psychology of Kundalini Yoga: Notes of the Seminar Given
in 1932 by C.G. Jung* (Princeton University Press, 1999), 107.

natural world in terms of types and categories of animals and plants—flora, fauna, and the numerous species and subspecies is a solar plexus chakra attribute. It is the cognitive processor and tends to use logic and reason to define reality.

This chakra has many attributes and tends to dominate the mind. Descartes said, "I think, therefore I am." This is a pure manipurism—we identify with our thoughts, opinions, ego, aversion, etc., and think that this is who we are.

When you think of the solar plexus chakra, think "separation and limitation." We make a sense of self out of our thoughts and wants and this separates us from others. Since the subjective self and the objective self are both illusions—that is, the true nature of reality is non-dual, subjectivity is always present in objectivity and vice versa—there is no contradiction in them both residing in the same chakra.

There is a saying in Spanish that points to this self-centrality. *En cada cabeza es un mundo.* In each head is a world. Samskaras here tend to increase the separating aspects and produce disengagement. The world shrinks because the mind becomes "tight" and grasping and we become overly self-conscious. Thus, the health of the solar plexus chakra determines how engaged we are with self, others, and life.

Thinking is an abstraction that separates from experience. The experience is the reality not the thought about the experience. When input from the physical senses (touching a hot surface, for example,) is turned into the thought ("This is hot!") that is a solar plexus chakra attribute. The experience of hot is in the body, but the thought of hot rises from the solar plexus chakra. It then wants to understand hot intellectually so it categorizes it in degrees and makes opposites. Hot is now not only a sensation reaction to an experience but also the opposite of cold. This process continues to: "How does something become hot? How can I heat something?" etc.

Although I discuss the negative aspects of the solar plexus chakra in this chapter, note that on the positive side, the strength aspects of a healthy solar plexus chakra are will, drive, courage, control, determination, and grit.

Orientation in Place and Time

This perspective placing the self as the center of everything enables us to orient ourselves in the world—me as separate from you and to be able to find our direction in the physical sense. "I am the center of the universe and every orientation point of the ten directions (the eight compass points plus up and down) is east, west, north, south, etc., of me. I am here and everything else is over there." Our viewpoint is always self-centered.

It is believed that animals that migrate, such as turtles and birds, use the magnetic poles as an orienting guide. Humans use this chakra in order to orient physically as well as orient us to our direction in life. We then use the other positive aspects such as drive and will to help get us there.

When this energy is "off," it will often manifest on both the psychological and physical levels. Not only can one become "lost in thought," but I often note that people who feel "lost" in the career or relationship areas sometimes have a difficult time orienting in the physical world. Donna, for example, is both confused about her direction in life and afraid to drive because she often gets lost. There is a general sense of being lost in one or another area of life

Abigail has said, "I am still trying to navigate relationships. It feels like a foreign land and I don't have the map that others do."

Linear thinking is just a method of orientation that helps us function on a day-to-day basis. The solar plexus chakra likes to use ideas to make things and then become attached to them. It makes past, present, and future and then, not satisfied with that, imposes a structure on it. Time is broken down into millenniums, centuries, decades, years, months, days, hours, minutes, and seconds. We *say* it is twelve o'clock, but there really is no twelve o'clock, there is only just now. In New York our three o'clock is California's twelve o'clock. If two people speak on the telephone in different time zones, they are both sharing the same moment even though their clocks differ. At every point on the face of the clock, it is only this moment. There is no past or future but only the present. Time is not linear and our circular-faced clocks clue us to that.

Like the subject/object duality, time is a construct used by the solar plexus chakra to help us function in life. We then use it to make schedules and plans. It is so useful to us that we fail to see that time is a construct and instead live in the illusion, thinking that it is real. The turn of the century and millennium in the year 2000 in the West is an example of how we come to believe the solar plexus chakra time illusion and make a big deal of something that is not real. Many anticipated a big positive or negative shift at the turn of the millennium. Many said, "Oh, something terrible is going to happen." But in reality there is no turn of the millennium; it is only an idea about time. In the Western world at the turn of the millennium we said it was the year 2000, in the Middle East they were up to 5760, in China they were up to 4698.

When there are significant samskaras here, one can be trapped in thoughts about the past or the future, usually with fear associated with it. Specifically, fear that something painful that happened in the past will happen again in the future. Paradoxically, those who fear the future the most often fail to plan for it. Time gets jumbled and one doesn't take the necessary steps such as putting money aside to secure a safe future. This is a good example of how samskaras produce difficult situations as one will have good reason to fear the future if there are no resources put aside.

Engagement

Many samskaras here create a shield of crystallized ego, fear, and rigid concepts—one becomes trapped in the thinking mind and disengaged from experience. There is an important point to be made about Traya and why it works. The psyche demands recognition of our experiences and their impact—not just thinking about them or talking about them from the surface mind or even with added emotion. Traya works because it moves one out of the thinking mind into the "experience mind" by reconnecting with the deep mind and the energy of the past experience. Traya moves us out of abstraction into reality.

The health of the solar plexus chakra determines how engaged we are with self, others, and life. Samskaras here actually contribute to an important coping mechanism in dealing with trauma by helping us control our emotions in difficult situations by distancing from them. Often so-called resilient people are operating from an overactive solar plexus chakra enabling them to control (or distance from) their feelings and environment in order to cope. Willpower is used to bear painful feelings. This is the "shutting down" of people out of touch with feelings and it becomes difficult to relate to them. Unfortunately, we cannot just decide to let go of a coping mechanism once the situation changes. When we live in uncomfortable situations growing up and feel we must be self-reliant, we retreat into the ego and it becomes unbalanced. Muriel saw this clearly while exploring the solar plexus chakra:

> ...I found myself in a home with tons of emotional turmoil, so I detached.

If we distance from ourselves, we distance from everything. Even our children with whom we want to be close will pick up on the distancing energy. If you are not in touch with your feelings, how can you be in touch with anyone else's? This feeling of separation moves us to spend too much time alone. It produces a sense of never really belonging and of being different and not able to "figure out" how to be happy.

Sara, while doing Traya, sees:

> ...I can't see what would fulfill me. I am still on the outside.
> ...Never really had actual feelings for a guy—that part of me doesn't work. It is all going on in my head not my heart.
> ...I have never inhabited my own life. Always reacting and never acting.

She realizes that she keeps a safe distance from people and will isolate at home many weekends, curling up with her books, because it feels easier than engaging with others. This fortifies her sense of isolation. She feels anxious and expresses the fear that if she lets her guard down, "there won't be anything there." We explored her anxious feelings and were led to the solar plexus chakra, where the following memory came up:

> ...*In seventh grade there was a boy who was very attractive. I was passed a note ostensibly from him that said, "Do you like me? I like you." I wrote yes and sent it back. He was football gorgeous and I was the fat girl with the glasses. He shared it and everyone laughed. I am afraid to open up and be vulnerable because I will be humiliated again.*
>
> *I am ashamed of being so naïve and falling for it. I built a wall—a crystalline artificial structure. I hold myself and my humor back. I am afraid to show myself.*

Sara's "crystalline" wall allowed her to numb her painful feelings. Human beings are very sensitive (not some but all) and situations like this, especially as a child, are shattering to the ego. Sara's feelings are pushed down and her trust in others is damaged. She asks me, "Why did this affect me so much?" I tell her that there are two big lies we tell both ourselves and others. One is "I didn't let it bother me," and the other is "Sticks and stones may break my bones, but names will never hurt me." As we have seen in our discussion of samskaras, we have no control over what bothers us or not. Is the situation out of resonance with the chakra? Yes, period. We can use our will to distance from the reaction, but that doesn't change the energetic impact. Her distancing wall helped her control her intense negative feelings when growing up. Now the wall itself is a problem preventing her from engaging fully with people, self, and life.

Distant significant others and not "fitting in" are some of the common causes of distancing energy. When we disengage from our feelings, we are not really alive. A sense of belonging is so important to healthy development. Katarina was ostracized in middle school and still feels like an "outsider":

> ...*I never worked at a job where I felt I belonged. I was not part of the office culture. I feel that I don't belong anywhere. I don't fit in.*

Ellen too has had social fear issues and has always struggled with not belonging:

> *...In college I did things that I didn't want to do in order to be-long. I dated a guy in college that I didn't really like so I wouldn't be alone any longer and would belong. He mistreated me and then avoided me.*

This last one is at least a quintuple solar plexus chakra whammy. First, she used willpower to push herself to do what she didn't want to. Second, she used alcohol to smooth the way. Third, she had to distance from herself to date him as a part of her knew he wasn't good for her. Fourth, she regrets these bad decisions. And even fifth, she was trying to relieve her isolation by taking action to "make" herself fit in more—control.

In summary, an unhealthy solar plexus chakra produces fear and tendencies to make self an end in itself. Since modern society values this over-intellectualized energy, it can be difficult to see the trap. The type A personality—self-sufficient, intellectual, willful, controlling, self-centered, selfish, and stressed—is becoming the common man or woman, a valued employee. Carl Jung, in describing the philosopher Nietzsche in the following quotation, provides a perfect example of a dissonant solar plexus chakra and the over-intellectualized disengaged person:

> Nietzsche had lost the ground under his feet because he possessed nothing more than the inner world of his thoughts—which, incidentally, possessed him more than he it. He was uprooted and hovered above the earth, and, therefore, he succumbed to exaggeration and irreality. For me, such irreality was the quintessence of horror, for I aimed, after all, at this world and this life. [11]

---

11. Paul Bishop, *The Dionysian Self: C.G. Jung's Reception of Friedrich Nietzsche* (Berlin; New York: Walter de Gruyter, 1995), 74.

When full engagement is absent from your life, it is impossible to imagine what it is like to have it. When this attribute is healed with Traya, fear and disengagement disappear and there is a profound shift to a better quality of life.

Control

Controlling feelings and hiding them from others for fear of embarrassment is a solar plexus chakra skill. It also helps us to remain in control in stressful situations by favoring the intellectual, problem-solving aspects of our minds. If we felt either overly controlled or a lack of control when growing up, we may try to control others and/or exhibit a lack of self-control. A child needs to feel that someone is in control but this must be balanced.

We are taught that in order to be successful, "you have to *make* it happen." Yes, we need drive, focus, and determination to get ahead, but we also must be able to read the subtle signs and realize when something has no energy—and not go in that direction. Fear leads one to want control. The rigidity of this stance also creates poor social skills. This tendency to be "in control" can become so entrenched that one develops compulsive thoughts or actions in order to feel in control. Lorna can't leave the house without checking the stove and faucets at least three times. Traya revealed:

> ...I am trying to prevent a disaster.

The flip side of control is overwhelmingness. She had been overwhelmed by several disasters in her home life growing up, including the death of a sibling. She often feels overwhelmed by the amount of work that she has to do every week. Her "control energy" is off and she flips back and forth between over control and overwhelm.

Focus

When unbalanced, one is distracted instead of focused. Too much thinking and worry interferes with focus and impacts the ability to learn. When there is lack of focus and distraction, there is also usually fear energy. Those with substantial fear as children report that it interfered with their ability to learn. Ellen reports that her anxiety interfered with her ability to learn in college:

> ...*I would read words and not compute what I read.*
> ...*I was barely making it through classes. I felt pushed to the side because of my difficulty with focus. I felt trapped.*
> ...*I was an English major and I had three books to read a week. It was overwhelming. I never figured out how to balance my time.*

(Note the four solar plexus chakra issues in one sentence—overwhelming, figure out, balance, and time). Her inability to focus and learn increased her stress, contributing to more samskaras being deposited and worsening her anxiety—like Lego blocks, building the fear level higher and higher.

Lack of focus is not always this dramatic or clear. June never realized she lacked focus, but after working with the solar plexus chakra, she saw that she was better able to focus on what she was doing. She reported that she watched an old movie she had seen before but was able to take it in as never before. Harry noticed that he always had a "vague consciousness on the edge of the music." He never really knew who was singing or what the song was about. Now he is more aware and hears the lyrics when songs are playing.

There is a pleasure in complete focus. When there are samskaras, we seek distraction to escape our problems or negative thoughts in our heads. We play video games or go to the movies and that helps get us "out of ourselves," and fear and worry fade temporarily.

Trust and Decision-Making

The solar plexus chakra's digestion of ideas, reality testing, and rational thinking all contribute to sound decision-making. The tendency in this chakra is to overvalue these aspects of decision-making and ignore our intuition. If there are more pros, we do "this," or if more cons, we do "that" instead.

> Frank: ...*I think I can control things by thinking them through—I am always in my head.*

Making good life decisions is crucial. If we go down a path that is not good for us in relationships or work, we will suffer, pile on more samskaras, and may never find our correct way. Some are stuck in jobs and careers they don't like because they were influenced by others or by "what made sense at the time." There is a tendency to try to "figure out" how to "make" things work out in the future. Sometimes we only feel the attraction or inclination to go in a certain direction but because we don't have a clear road map with all of the twists and turns to come clearly outlined and can't see how we can "make" it happen, we abandon the idea. Ana was in this predicament. "I am of two minds," she said, "so I don't know what to do."

The truth is that life doesn't work by pros and cons and clear road maps. We can't figure out the future, we can only proceed decision by decision. We can never know the opportunities that will appear if we go down a certain path. We do know, however, that it is likely no opportunities will appear in the field or area that we are attracted to if we don't start on that path.

Most of us are familiar with the regret of looking back at a period in our lives when we made a bad choice or decision and we can acknowledge that "something didn't feel right" about that choice at that time and wish that we had trusted that feeling. So there is something in us that tells us when something is not "right." The ability to connect with this and trust it is the secret to an authentic life. However, for so many, an unbalanced solar plexus chakra gets in the way of heeding these messages and instead we second guess ourselves.

Sara once said, "With my previous relationship, I went into my head and disconnected from my heart. I was analyzing everything."

Now when she starts a new relationship, she doesn't trust her own feelings: "How do I know I am not just infatuated?"

Lack of structure, or too much structure, growing up can lead to difficulties with decision-making. If there is no structure then one is "hanging out there" on one's own and often making poor decisions. Or when there is too much structure and decisions are made for us, we don't trust ourselves to make decisions either. Both are fear provoking. A history of bad decisions creates a fear of repeating them. A history of being controlled leads to a lack of self-trust, fear of making a mistake, and trying to control the future. A history of peer rejection and/or bullying leads to a shattered ego and lack of self-trust.

Clarity and Reality Testing

It is paradoxical that reality testing is in the solar plexus chakra—the great illusion maker that "makes" duality. If someone says that there are aliens in the bedroom, your knowledge about that person, reason, memory, intellect, and common sense kick in and you don't assume that it is true. All kinds of crazy information comes over the airwaves and online, but if we have good reality testing, we can say, most likely, that isn't true. The solar plexus chakra fear and imbalance can get in the way of reality testing and one will think the worst when there is no evidence for it. One overreacts and lacks objectivity. "I did bad on one test; therefore, I am never going to be able to achieve my goals in life."

The rational approach of the solar plexus chakra doesn't usually work when interpersonal relations are concerned because relationships don't operate on that plane. Other solar plexus chakra aspects such as the tendency to grasp and cling can interfere with living in relationship reality. You may know on a rational level that things are not working for you, but on the emotional level it is hard to let go and move on. Or you may not be able to "put two and two together" and see the picture of the impossibility of the relationship clearly.

Confusing messages when growing up create lingering confusion in the mind.

Matt often complains that it is hard for him to "figure things out." "I am not sure of what is real." Traya revealed:

> …I was confused because with my father I couldn't do anything right and with my mother I couldn't do anything wrong. There was no realistic input so I can't feel that I have confidence in what I am doing. I am left with confusion about my direction.

If, when growing up, your sense of reality is questioned or dismissed, then these attributes will be compromised. Helen had difficulty seeing the reality in her romantic relationship in which her boyfriend was undependable and never put her first. She had a tendency to focus on what she was doing wrong (exploding with rage) rather than her boyfriend's dysfunctional behavior that set her off. She brought in a letter her mother sent to her when she was sixteen years old. Some excerpts:

—…how deeply you hurt me…

—You are not there when I need your help the most.

—Your main interest is yourself.

Her mother turned reality upside down as it was Helen who was hurt and abandoned and it is her mother who is the responsible selfish one. Now Helen cannot perceive the reality of her current situation either—she keeps the focus on her reaction to her boyfriend's selfish behavior and feels wrong.

When the solar plexus chakra is healthy, one is able to process situations at the moment and understand them clearly and intelligently.

Note: The solar plexus chakra is not involved with significant disconnects from reality such as delusions, paranoia, and hallucinations, and that is why evidence, logic, and reason do not work in convincing someone of something obvious to everyone else, e.g., the television news anchor you never met is not in love with you.

Judgment

Good judgment is a positive trait of the solar plexus chakra. If exposed to judgment and criticism from others when growing up, an "inner critic" will develop and we may judge others and ourselves just as harshly. This voice can feel like it is part of us rather than the pain body and we then feel guilty for having this tendency. Judgment often involves comparison.

Ania: "I don't like competition because I always lose."

…I was compared to everyone as a child by my mother. You are not social like so and so. My mother wasn't either and I get it from her but I was blamed.

...In college looks were so important. Now I feel as though people like me because of external things.

Indeed, although she is very attractive, she often mentions that she will never get a guy because she has gained a few pounds or she is not bubbly enough.

A tendency to judge is another limiting and isolating force. Our likes and dislikes narrow our world. Sammy was new in town, unemployed, and feeling isolated. I suggested that he volunteer at the LGBT community center. He said, "Oh, only lost people go there." He says of his boyfriend's friends, "Roy's friends are slouches. I can't relate to them." This example shows clearly how this solar plexus chakra tendency contributes to isolation. One of the beauties of Traya is that you don't have to be told you are judgmental and feel judged. When we explored the solar plexus chakra, Sammy received his education directly from the deep mind:

...Judgment and criticism keep me separate.

After we worked with this judgment energy, he opened up and went to the LGBT center and made friends and connections there. Later, he was also able to enjoy the company of his boyfriend's friends.

Opposite to being judgmental is not trusting one's own judgment. Sara said, "My experiences have eroded my trust in my judgment. I spent the first half of my life doing the wrong moves. I opened up at the wrong time. I stood up for myself at the wrong time and didn't stand up for myself at the right time. I had no compass. No north star."

Willpower

Willpower is one of the "driving forces" of the solar plexus chakra. This chakra produces a healthy drive toward accomplishment of goals by keeping us interested in our goals and determined to achieve them. An overuse of willpower such as "surviving by willpower alone," as Millie put it, can produce a tendency to engage in "battles of the wills."

Millie has lots of "fighting relationships" with coworkers, family members, and romantic partners. She vehemently relates her conversations with them—they didn't do this, or they did that. Her chakra is so "tight" it is physically uncomfortable and she feels a constant knot in her stomach. She is in a perpetual "battle of the wills" with the people around her. She says she wants to be free of it and to bring into her life an engaged and dependable man. You can guess what we found when we did Traya here.

…My father is always picking fights. He is resentful toward my mother.

She speaks about her father with the same vehemence she displays when talking about the people in her life who provoke her. When she describes her long-term relationship with a man that ended, it sounds like it was a constant battle of the wills and let downs. She says she doesn't want men to fight with yet she somehow finds the ones who also want to battle.

The opposite of willfulness is too much "surrender energy." Remember that an unbalanced chakra can have too much of an attribute or not enough of it. Judith complains of always giving in to others—paying for shoddy work and giving in to her husband too much. Traya revealed:

…My older brother was so wrong, but you couldn't reason with him. You have to do what he wants or noisy violence doesn't stop. …You cannot make him wrong—no choice but to surrender.

Willpower is also an important aspect of delayed gratification and choice. When it is out of balance, too much or too little, there often is impulsivity, compulsive behaviors and/or a lack of drive.

Courage
Fearlessness is the prize of a healthy solar plexus chakra. The generic definition of courage is "firmness of spirit that meets danger without fear." A common issue here is fear of the future. This makes sense since the solar plexus chakra creates our sense of time, and if there is

fear energy present, it will sometimes take that form as the solar plexus chakra pulls us into the past or future. One may say that all fear is fear of the future as one is consciously or unconsciously anticipating that something bad is going to happen. Ellen was fearful she would not find a satisfying career. The following surfaced when we explored this "fear energy" at the solar plexus chakra:

> …*My grandfather always said, "Work gets in the way of life." Most people that I know hate their jobs and are unhappy. I don't want my work life to be like that.*

Financial fear is one of the most debilitating fears. There is a sense of always living on the edge of disaster. Judith, who grew up in a single-parent family in the South, is fearful of her online clothing business failing as it has been slow of late:

> …*Once as a teenager, the family was so broke. My mother took out the chest where she kept the cash and showed me that there was no money in it. I was afraid that the family would split up and I could not think of losing her.*
> …*My mother tried to start different businesses but they all failed. She was devastated and I felt helpless.*

Now she is back in this situation again (inside/outside maxim), only she is the business owner. While abundance is a heart chakra attribute, financial fear appears here too because it is also connected to several solar plexus issues—focus on future (not having enough in the immediate future), fear, lack of control, dependence on problem-solving (how can I make it different), and imbalance (living on the edge is an extreme situation).

Other chakras can also have fear energy—for example, the fear of rejection in the heart chakra or the fear of being seen in the throat chakra—but the bulk of material producing fear will be in the solar plexus chakra.

Myra said, "But isn't everyone living in fear? This is a dangerous world. How can you not be anxious all of the time?" I explained the difference between "genuine" fear and "mind" fear. Genuine fear is based on real external situations occurring in the moment or are clearly about to occur that are dangerous in some way. It is a tool for keeping ourselves safe. Mind fear is an internalized sense of fear and worry that occurs even when there is no impending danger. It is caused by an imbalanced solar plexus chakra resulting from exposure to fearful situations in the past. The "fight-or-flight switch" is stuck in the on position. When one is stuck in this mode, there is no space for self-reflection; there is just reaction. Yes, there is danger in the world, but it is not constantly on the mind. It will rise up and it will also re-cede. If I am driving and am cut off and almost crash into another car, I get really scared. After it is over and everyone is safe, I calm down and the fear recedes and I move on with my day. With mind fear the fear is always present regardless of the absence of a dangerous situa-tion—receding only slightly and also getting worse at times.

Fairness and Justice
A good symbol for this chakra is the blind justice statue with the bal-anced scales, as it creates our sensitivity to fairness and justice. If you want to see this in action, just spend time around children whose an-tennas always seem to be up around this issue. Alice said:

> ...Children know injustice, and not to be able to respond to it is hard.

Ellen feels a sense of injustice because the things that she liked were never encouraged:

> ...Academics were a struggle, but creative things were easy—I have a self that is brushed aside. I am put down for things that I can't do and the things that I can are not recognized.

Balance
The justice symbol with the balanced scales is appropriate also be-cause the solar plexus chakra also governs the balance of the mind. When there is extreme excitement or fear, the balance is thrown off and there can be an "addiction" to excitement or fear. For example,

Marion experienced extreme emotions in her tumultuous relationship with her father. Now, in relationships with men, she believes they are not satisfactory because they lack intensity. She has a secret crush on her boss who is married. He pays her a lot of attention and she interprets this as him feeling the same way about her. Secret relationships provide a thrill and the intensity she is looking for. His unavailability also keeps her safe from an actual romantic relationship with genuine closeness that she is not ready to allow into her life. Living in fantasy is a solar plexus chakra condition that consists of supplying thrills that are not available in ordinary life.

Violet feels a sudden sick feeling in her stomach, "a frustrated, doomed feeling," when her husband starts to loudly argue with her. The moment beforehand, everything is fine. When we worked with this, the following came up:

> ...One little thing can turn the tables.
> ...I was sitting with my friends on the porch when I was eight, and we had one of those magic eight balls and were having fun with it. My teenaged brother came out and I said, "Jack, try this; you can see your future." He took it and threw it to the sidewalk and it smashed. He did things like that often.
> ...Unexpected hostility that comes out of nowhere. I can't let down my guard.

This type of memory often arises in an unbalanced solar plexus chakra. Hostile energy coming at you from out of nowhere when people's reactions are extreme and not congruent with the situation.

An unbalanced solar plexus chakra inflates the ego and produces self-importance. One may fantasize about future achievements and have grandiose ideas about success or flip between self-aggrandizement and self-debasement. Both are isolating and uncomfortable mind states.

We all deride the narcissistic person but we fail to realize that they are trapped in this mind state—it is not a personality defect but a samskaric state of mind. Retreating into the safety of the ego (a "normal" reaction in stressful circumstances) for self-protection, the ego becomes inflated and egotistic consciousness dominates. Sheila said, "I am the most important person in the world because no one made me important in their world."

Another person said, "I don't want to ride a monorail above everyone else."

Ania often overreacts when upset:

> ...*Mother exaggerated little things—almost out of gas, she was hysterical.*

This imbalance energy in the solar plexus chakra leads to the tendency to look at life through a "black or white" filter with little or no hues. One fails to see the nuances: e.g., everything is OK or it is a catastrophe, or I need to be apologizing or I am obnoxious. Black and white thinking also leads to intolerance and an imbalance in the problem-solving tendency of this chakra. Simplistic and extreme solutions are embraced.

Drive and Vitality

In a healthy solar plexus chakra, drive helps us to move forward toward the achievement of our goal or goals. On the other hand, one can become compulsively driven, fiercely competitive, and willing to do anything regardless of the impact on self or others. Or if underactive, one may tend to drift. The black and white thinking described earlier was one of the factors affecting Steve's drive:

> ...*Difficult to find direction—no options. Can only see big and little picture. Everything in between is left out.*

Ego-centered drive is a symptom of a samskaric solar plexus chakra. "I want to be president of the company so people will see how great I am." This is different than the more authentic drive that is involved with efforts toward self-actualization. Authentic drive has strength and vitality yet is not egocentric and one doesn't need to push or make things happen.

Responsibility

The solar plexus chakra's attribute of control and decision-making contribute to a healthy sense of responsibility. This too can become imbalanced, and over-responsibility or irresponsibility can appear with either grandiosity and/or guilt usually present.

Sheila cannot understand why she feels so responsible for her adult son and her difficulty in letting go of taking care of him financially although he is approaching thirty. Traya revealed:

> ...I feel guilty because I wasn't the best parent when he was young. So busy with work and being a single parent and not providing him with a good father figure. My stuff just got in the way.

On the other hand, many have difficulty taking responsibility for their behaviors and failing to understand their impact on others. Ryan found many reasons to place blame for his difficulties on others in his daily life. He could only see how he was being wronged. Again, when one is blind to their own shortcomings, Traya can gently highlight these defects without one feeling judged or misunderstood. Traya revealed:

> ...My mother was always talking about who was wronging her.

He saw how he picked up this lack of responsibility and this blaming of others' energy from his relatives.

Calm, Ease, and Flexibility

When the solar plexus chakra is healthy and balanced, there is a sense of calm, ease, and flexibility. One can readily "go with the flow" without needing to control or direct. All of the positive aspects of this chakra combine to make one feel confident about the future and navigate life without stress. Emotions flow freely, when good things happen one can be happy. When bad things happen one can be sad. Emotions are balanced and one does not become excessively excited about ideas and plans nor does one encounter extreme situations in one's life. Life itself becomes a flow without fear or the need to "make" things happen.

Release Chakra (Mukta)

- **Location:** pit of stomach
- **Function:** release

Mukta and abhaya (the secondary chakra that lies below mukta) are unique in that they border each other instead of lie between two primary chakras, as the other secondary chakras do. Mukta lies between the fearless chakra (abhaya) and the solar plexus chakra. The release chakra provides the ability to completely let go and relax into experience. A helpful image when contemplating it is either an open hand (healthy) or closed (unhealthy) fist. This chakra holds the tension in the body created by a fearful solar plexus chakra. Once when working with Sheila and the release chakra, the following appeared:

…I need to let go of being in charge.

This is a scary thing to her as she has already let go of so much control energy from the solar plexus chakra. This requires a lot of trust. We found a memory preventing release:

…I always felt as though there was no one in charge at home growing up. I needed to hold on.

A lot of negative energy comes out and she realizes how she has been holding this energy back and her entire body relaxes. The positive imprint brings in "freedom."

When this chakra relaxes from the Traya work, the result is palpable. I do not recommend approaching the release chakra directly, but rather wait to be led there in the Traya process. In the example prior, Sheila had years of Traya work behind her and was ready to completely let go and be fully present. This cannot be forced.

••• EXERCISE: TRAYA PRACTICE AT THE ••• SOLAR PLEXUS CHAKRA (MANIPURA)

Grounding

Ground by sitting up straight, focusing on the soles of your feet, and breathing in and out of the tertiary chakras in the feet.

Following Memories Technique

This is another deep mind–guided technique, but instead of thinking of an issue in your current life, you are going to think of a negative memory that you are already aware of. Let's say you were criticized by a teacher and embarrassed in front of your classmates, for example. This incident stands out in your mind. Focus on your body and ask, "Where in me is the energy related to this?" You feel a sensation at the solar plexus chakra. You then continue with the Traya steps.

> **Step 1: Focus**—Keep your attention on the solar plexus chakra and breathe in and out gently.
>
> **Step 2: Surface**—You already have the memory so you don't need to surface it. After you begin the release process with this memory, you can then ask, "What other memories are here?"
>
> **Step 3: Release**—Continuously add to the outflow of negative energy memory by memory. After you are finished surfacing memories for this session, let all of the negative energy go out and wait until the outflow stops.
>
> **Step 4: Replace and Imprint**—Visualize positive energy coming in (rays from the sun) and taking up the space that was taken up by the negative energy that went out. Ask, "What is this positive energy bringing in with it?" Note the words that appear in your mind.
>
> **Step 5: Scene from Nature (Optional)**—Breathe in and out while focusing attention on the solar plexus chakra and let a scene from nature appear in your mind. Note if the fire element is strong. (See the list of chakra elements in chapter 2.)

Finish by grounding again.

••• EXERCISE: TRAYA PRACTICE AT THE ••• RELEASE CHAKRA (MUKTA)

You use the following memories technique we just reviewed. You remember your father giving one of your toys away that you weren't ready to let go of, for example, and you are led to mukta, located right in the pit of your stomach between abhaya (fearless) and the solar plexus chakra. Next is to continue with the Traya practice. You ground by breathing in and out of the soles of your feet.

Step 1: Focus—Keep your attention on mukta and breathe in and out gently.

Step 2: Surface—You already have the memory so you don't need to surface it. After you begin the release process with this memory, you can then ask, "What other memories are here?"

Step 3: Release—Keep adding to the chain of negative energy going out. When it stops, proceed to step 4.

Step 4: Replace and Imprint—Visualize positive energy coming in (rays from the sun) and taking up the space that was taken up by the negative energy that went out. Ask, "What is this positive energy bringing in with it?" Note the words that appear in your mind.

There is no scene from nature step with the secondary chakras. Finish by grounding.

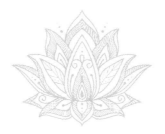

Chapter 9

THE HEART CHAKRA (ANAHATA) AND THE SELF-ESTEEM CHAKRA (VAJRAHRIDAYA)

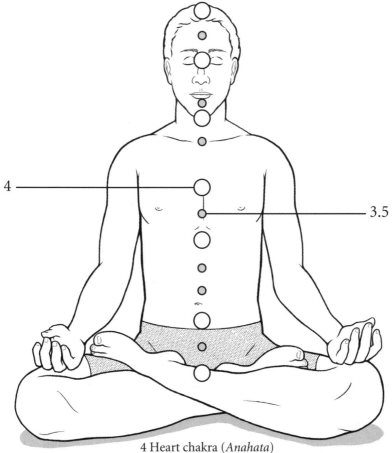

4 Heart chakra (*Anahata*)
3.5 Self-esteem chakra (*Vajrahridaya*)

Figure 9: Fourth Chakra

Anahata, the Heart Chakra

- **Function:** connection to self, others, nature, life, spirit
- **Attributes:** love, knowledge, inspiration, trust, hope, joie de vivre, enthusiasm, empathy, confidence, desire, abundance, generosity, fullness, truth, passion, forgiveness, compassion, happiness
- **Attribute paradox:** "I can't trust my heart."
- **Common issues in anahata:** sadness, loneliness, lack of enthusiasm, confidence, or trust

A healthy heart chakra produces an abiding joy in being alive and a reverence for nature. It makes life worth living by connecting us to self, others, nature, and spirit. It provides a sense of fullness and buoyancy similar to the uplifted feeling we have when walking in nature and we come upon a beautiful landscape.

Our language reveals an intuitive understanding of the positive aspects of the heart chakra located in the center of the chest—"My heart leapt." "My heart is full." When the heart chakra is in its healthiest state, life takes on a rosy glow and there is a sense of joie de vivre and possibility. A samskaric heart chakra produces sadness, loneliness, and emptiness and if very samskaric, depression and hopelessness. The heart chakra is one of the organs where the subtle body energy can sometimes be "felt" and, again, our language reveals an intuitive association: "heavy heart," "heartbreak," "my heart sank." With rejecting experiences, contracting, heavy, or squeezing sensations are felt in the chest contrary to the fullness and expansive warmth of loving experiences.

In the heart chakra, we leave the self-centered I-consciousness of the solar plexus chakra and step into "not two" consciousness—we move from duality to oneness. In the solar plexus chakra, we see ourselves as the center of the universe, and in the heart chakra we have a sense of oneness with everything.

The heart chakra element is air—the breath of life. It connects to the energy of life and the energy of spirit. The word "spirit" is derived from the Latin "spiritus," which means both breath and spirit.

We all need to be respected, heard, understood, and to feel that we matter to the people in our lives. This empathic attunement strengthens the heart chakra and we feel a healthy sense of connection to and trust in others. When we feel loved and cared for, we are able to love and care for ourselves and others. As Francine put it, "Attention is the first currency."

The opposite too holds true—when someone is not fully connected to themselves, they cannot fully connect to others. Connection requires interaction, engagement, and understanding. A parent may really try, but the deep mind cannot be fooled and it will pick up on any lack of "connection energy" and it will have an impact. Maybe the child will see that you are not really listening or fully engaged or you don't quite love yourself fully, or you do not have passion for life and will pick up "disconnection energy" as a samskara or samskaras. You can't pretend to really connect—either you have "connection energy" or you don't.

Sara felt a lack of connection to others, so she tried to make up for it. This came up while working at the heart:

> …*My superpower is to be a chameleon and make everyone feel like I find them interesting. I am not connecting—I am just stroking their ego.*

Marilyn was working on her lack of self-confidence. With Traya she realized that although her parents were enthusiastically supportive, it didn't ring true:

> …*I couldn't have been so wonderful at everything they said that I was. I knew I couldn't believe them or trust them so I didn't know what to believe about myself.*

It is lack of connection with significant others, loss, hostility, betrayal, abandonment, and disappointment in people that most impacts the heart chakra.

Daniela generally focuses on the negative aspects of what is going on around her. She believes that people are trying to "get one over" on her. She carries a "fighting energy" as she often gets into minor scrapes with people and is in a relationship where there is frequent fighting. These memories came up at her heart chakra:

> ...*I took part in every extracurricular activity in school and often stayed over at friends' houses to escape the constant fighting at home.*
> ...*My best friend moved away when I was fourteen years old and then my aunt died.*
> ...*I felt alone without being alone. There was a general vibe of loss and melancholy weighing on me over the years.*

Fighting is a disconnecting energy and so is loss. These were both samskaric in Daniela's heart chakra. To experience loss, there doesn't need to be a death. Even if the person is in your life or in your home, if they are inaccessible, then that is a loss of connection energy. Daniela's fighting family was inaccessible and now her husband is alternatingly angry and shutting down. It is not that they choose to be unavailable; they are like Sara—unable to pull off connection because of their own wounded hearts. Sara struggles with her need for love and her conviction that she is not worthy of it. While working with the Traya techniques at the heart, she said:

> ...*I feel that I am living just on the surface with people. I feel like no one is closer than arm's length. I want to access a deeper level of connection but I am afraid that I am not there.*

We explored this limitation:

> ...*Every time I feel accessed by others I get defensive. I am never comfortable being in the regard of someone.*

Then we explored the origin of this defensiveness:

> ...*I am articulate because my inner landscape is words. I describe things because I cannot feel them.*
> ...*With friends I was low in the pecking order. When I was myself it was so bad.*

...I always walked around thinking they were right. How could so many people be wrong?

...My adoption was my original wound—unwanted. And everything just built on that.

...I always feared my adopted parents didn't really want me. I wasn't theirs.

Confidence and Trust

In his book *The Speed of Trust*, Stephen M. R. Covey observes the importance of trust in all aspects of life.

> There is one thing that is common to every individual, relationship, team, family, organization, nation, economy, and civilization throughout the world—one thing which, if removed, will destroy the most powerful government, the most successful business, the most thriving economy, the most influential leadership, the greatest friendship, the strongest character, the deepest love.... That one thing is trust.[12]

Just as important is self-trust. The heart chakra's self-trust helps guide us through life. As noted, this develops from empathic authentic connections and a sense of safety with others.

The opposite of trust is distrust or paranoia. We are paranoid when we have an abiding sense or suspicion that people will harm us in some way. Sara had this: "I expect to walk into a room and people will whisper negative things. Kids did that in school."

Kara is attending grad school interviews at three institutions. She is dreading the part of the process where she sits down with a group of professors and answers their questions. In anticipation, her heart beats rapidly and "I almost can't breathe." She says she has prepared well and can't understand why she is distressed beyond normal interview jitters. We wanted to clear the way for a successful interview. We did Traya at the heart.

---

12. Stephen M.R. Covey with Rebecca R. Merrill, *The Speed of Trust: The One Thing That Changes Everything* (New York: Free Press, 2006), 3.

...When I was a teenager I fell off my bike and broke my arm. I had to call my mom to come and get me and take me to the doctor. Instead of concern, she was yelling, "Why aren't you more careful? Now I have to drop what I am doing and take you to the doctor." It becomes all about her and she unleashes her dragon anger. Whatever you are going through is nothing. I finally learned to stop going to her.

When you can't trust your own parents to be there for you, you project that distrust on to other people—particularly authority figures. Not only did her mother abandon her emotionally in her time of need, but she also lashed out at her. The resulting imprint is that you cannot trust people to understand you and that something bad will happen when you are in a vulnerable position with people. Confidence and trust are interdependent. We must trust others to have confidence in them and we must trust ourselves to have confidence in ourselves. Kara's "trust energy" is damaged so she can't trust herself to do a good job even though she knows the material well. She can't trust the professors to be pleasant and supportive. She can't trust life in the sense of knowing that everything will work out for the best. So she is afraid. She felt better after the session for several reasons: First, she was able to understand where this free-floating fear was coming from; second, at the end of the exploration when bringing in positive energy, two words appeared in her mind—"fearlessness and confidence"—and they brought tears to her eyes. Most importantly, by surfacing this distrust energy she now has less of it in her mind to cause fear and interfere with the interview process and her interactions with the interviewers. This dynamic with her mother was intense and chronic, so it will take some more work to completely heal it, but she is on her way. The interview went well and she later received her acceptance letter into the graduate program of her choice.

The relationship with a therapist is particularly beneficial in healing the heart chakra. Positive imprints counter the negative ones when the therapist understands her and she feels safety in her vulnerability without judgment or criticism. She has a place where it is "all about her." With both a healing relationship and the Traya work, she is well on her way to healing her heart chakra and activating its positive functions.

As trust, especially self-trust, is the key to maneuvering through life, I am providing another example of how trust energy becomes damaged and of the destructive results of that damage. This is an example from the memoir *Holy Hell* by Gail Tredwell:

> In my youth I had been a loyal friend and had gone out of my way to please. I never gave up on friendships even when the loyalty I displayed was far from reciprocated. I had one girlfriend in particular who was fine when it was just the two of us, but when another girl came into the picture, she would turn on me. One day the three of us were out having coffee and I briefly left the table for a bathroom visit. Upon return I began sipping my coffee, and the sight of that sent my friend and her accomplice into a fit of hysterical laughter. I later learned that the new girl had spat in my drink. … Growing up I experienced many similar incidents, and I sometimes felt so lonely and dejected that I would head to the nearby park and play on the swings as I shed tears. … Despite my broken heart I didn't have it in me to be mean in return, let alone to stand up for myself.[13]

She also describes a lack of connection to her parents and siblings at home. Thus, she was vulnerable and energetically "primed" for abuse in the external world. In not standing up for herself, she abandoned herself—another heart chakra wound. The abuse came from her "friends" and later, as she describes in her book, abuse from a guru to whom she had devoted her life. She wonders why she continued to abandon herself in her relationship with the guru and stuck around for twenty years. When trust energy is off, you can also trust the wrong people too fast because you don't trust yourself to know who to trust.

---

13. Gail Tredwell, *Holy Hell: A Memoir of Faith, Devotion, and Pure Madness* (Maui: Wattle Tree Press, 2013), 46–47.

Trust and love go hand in hand and if we are not trusted we will not feel loved. Marla feels that her distrustful husband doesn't love her:

...He doesn't trust me to have friends—I might cheat. He has missed the essence of me and doesn't know me.

At some point in working with the heart chakra, the issue of man's inhumanity to man is raised. When I worked with Francine at the heart chakra, the following came up:

...I want to believe in the basic goodness of people, but that is like a trap door. No hope that people will ever stop hurting each other.

Indeed it is a vicious circle; samskaras in the solar plexus and heart chakras create states of mind that drive people to justify hurting each other, and then new samskaras are created that then drive more hurt. It is urgent that we heal these energies in ourselves and free our positive energy to contribute to a healthier humanity.

Love

The sun transmits most of its energy in the green part of the visible spectrum where the heart chakra resonates. Therefore, it can be said that love is the dominant force in the solar system if not the universe. Love is an energy like every other state of mind. If we are loved as children, our love energy is strong and we feel self-love as well.

Jane has many people who like her and want to be around her as she has a good sense of humor and is attractive and considerate. Her abiding feeling that keeps her from closeness with others or herself is her lack of self-love. Her belief is that "people don't like me and I am incapable of connecting." Traya at the heart revealed the following:

...My parents didn't like me. They treated me with disdain and annoyance. I didn't do anything right. Everything about me is repulsive.
...Love can flip into hate.

She believes that she can only be worthy if someone else loves her, but if they know her they won't love her despite a lot of evidence to the contrary. It is a trap that keeps her disconnected from people and supports her abiding sense of unworthiness.

When one feels important to significant others, one feels loved. Donna was under-employed but was unable to muster the effort to seek work more on her level:

> ...My job helps me to hate myself. I reject myself because I have been rejected by my father my whole life.

Inez grew up in a divorced family. Both parents remarried when she was nine. She is having difficulty finding a loving relationship:

> ...I feel like my father is just not that into me. He moved to another state with his new family after the breakup and when I wanted to be more included he would say, "You should be here more." Like it was up to me.
> ...He always bitched and moaned that he was not spending enough time with me, but when I visited he would leave me alone.
> ...My grandmother would always visit my aunt and not us. I felt that we were the back-burner people.

Once the impact of the lack of parental love (or ability to demonstrate it) is understood, one can feel stuck. "How can I ever heal if I can never get that love from them of which I see they are incapable of giving?" The good news is that we don't need to get the love from outside anymore. We just need to remove the samskaras so that the love energy inherent in the heart can bloom and we can feel the fullness and joy that comes with it abiding in our consciousness. Then we love ourselves and all beings and we will have better loving relationships in our lives.

Compassion

As our heart heals and we have a clearer understanding of why people suffer, compassion arises for those with heavy hearts and fearful minds. We have some distance from our own solar plexus chakra's suffering and see how easily it trapped us. We realize that most of the problems human beings have with each other come from negative samskaras in the heart chakra and the solar plexus chakra and the resulting disconnection energy. We see that human beings are wired for love and compassion and that what is in us also permeates the universe. This is truly miraculous and answers Einstein's question, "Is the universe friendly?"

Self-compassion takes the form of self-care. That means that we do everything we can to stay healthy through exercise, diet, and lifestyle. We take care of health issues without putting them off. We take steps to resolve difficulties in relationships and stand up for ourselves when necessary. We do these things for several reasons but primarily because we want to feel better.

One of the often encountered wounds at the heart is self-abandonment related to not standing up for ourselves:

Ellen:...*I put up with mean friends.*

Joe:...*Kids in school insulted me and I didn't respond.*

When we have compassion for ourselves, we make sure that we stand up for ourselves because we know that we will feel better.

Forgiveness

As we increase our connection energy, forgiveness naturally appears because you cannot feel connected and still hold resentment. Remember that this is a process of healing that is driven by truth. People sometimes too soon say, "I forgive him/her." This is just an idea that is not backed up by real forgiveness energy. They have not healed their wounds in the heart chakra so cannot really forgive deeply in their hearts—only in their heads. I have heard it said that "premature forgiveness is like putting icing on a burnt cake." On the other hand, when true forgiveness (the heart chakra attribute) arises as one progresses with Traya, it is most welcome.

Sheila had a distant and painful relationship with her mother who could sometimes be cruel. She is elderly now and Sheila after a visit said, "It is a great gift to feel unconditional love for my mother. Taking her out and spending time with her, I no longer want something from her and she can no longer hurt me. I can see her beyond her wounds and I feel my open heart where it was always closed tight. It is a true joy."

The other side of this is when people sometimes feel they are blaming their parents unfairly and don't want to "dump" on them. My response is that it is truth that heals and it is true that they were wounded by some of their parents' behaviors even if their parents didn't mean to hurt them. You cannot have healing without accepting the truth. Then you can let go and reconnect with them in a new and deeper way.

Abundance and Generosity

The heart chakra connects us to life. Saving money is a life-affirming behavior because we are trusting in a future for ourselves and we care enough about ourselves to be responsible with our resources—this enhances our abundance. This is done without clinging as trust in life encourages generosity. We trust that there is enough and that as abundance flows toward us we don't have to squeeze our fists shut but rather open our hands wide. All of the heart chakra attributes bring joy, and generosity is one of the most pleasurable. Generosity is a sign of freedom.

Abundance comes from healthy heart chakra energy that is beyond the solar plexus chakra's limited perspective of grasping and clinging. When the heart energy is healthy, we are connected to the exuberant abundance of nature and generous, limitless spirit. Selfless desire replaces craving and we desire what is best for both ourselves and others. If we are connected to ourselves, we take care of ourselves, and then we have abundant health, we eat well, we don't smoke or drink to excess, we do yoga and meditation, and we don't do things that are unhealthy. This is not a willpower issue. We eat healthy because it is good for us and makes us feel good. We find our true work, which we love, and earn money too so we are doubly happy. A healthy heart chakra attracts positive situations—we are connected to more people and have more opportunity. We trust ourselves and, therefore, make the best choices.

When we live authentically, we have the support of the universe and we find that we always have what we need in both quality relationships and material abundance.

When we have authentic abundance generated by positive energy within, it does not contribute to a disconnection from others who don't have as much. Raina came from a wealthy family. Her father's unbalanced relationship to abundance and lack of authentic connection produced samskaras in her heart chakra:

> …*I felt the hypocrisy in the home. Father was a business mogul and his thing was how he had achieved more than his family— better than others didn't make sense. He was constantly comparing plus or minus.*

Her father had abundance but it wasn't authentic. It didn't come from the positive heart chakra attribute, and, therefore, he used it to buoy himself up at the expense of others—a behavior resulting from negative samskaras in both the heart and solar plexus chakras.

This is an example of a phenomenon I call "empty opulence." There is plenty of money and status but a significant lack of the connection energy that one really needs—leaving one with a sense of emptiness in the heart.

The solar plexus chakra too needs to be healed or it may interfere with our generosity and thus with the flow. Its clinging, grasping, overly rational, and limited perspective can get in the way. For example, when the earthquake devastated Haiti in 2010, the destruction was overwhelming. I heard someone say, "Giving money to Haiti is like throwing good money down a hole. There are so many problems they can never be fixed." The overactive, problem-solving, rational mind drowned out the heart energy. So we really have to understand our minds and how imbalances impact not only us but also the world.

Desire and Passion

The heart wants what it wants; do it with all your heart; devote your heart to it; wholehearted; my heart was not in it; in my heart of hearts… These are some of the terms that reveal an intuitive association of desire and passion with the heart.

The wanting in the heart comes from our deepest desire. Doing something to one's "heart's content" provides a deep inner satisfaction. The heart chakra moves us to live wholeheartedly. It gives us the strength of purpose to self-actualize.

Tela realized that she is focused more on what she doesn't want than what she wants. Her wanting energy is off:

… I was never allowed to have any wants growing up. The ones I did have weren't fulfilled.

Ellen's artistic abilities were discouraged as a child while she was encouraged to focus on academics:

…Nothing that I ever wanted was ever acknowledged. No one ever wanted me to be myself.

She is now an adult but is still afraid to acknowledge her talents and her desires. Her deep mind is encouraging her to follow her heart and do what she really wants—creative pursuits to bring art back into her life.

Violet fears that it is futile to want things. Traya revealed that her brother and niece died before their last wishes could be fulfilled— each wanted to go on a cruise before they died. Her brother was in a difficult marriage and once said to Violet, "I don't want to be with her until I die." He was.

Violet once told me, "My mother didn't want to be fat and play bingo either. I don't want to be like them. I want to get the few things that I want. I want to help people. I feel that is my purpose."

Aesthetic Sense

The desire for beauty is one of the most basic human desires. When we have the resources, we make ourselves and our surroundings more beautiful. Beauty uplifts the heart because the nature of the world is beauty and we connect to it in the heart chakra. If we are forced to live in an area that is not beautiful, there will be a negative effect on this chakra. When we encounter beauty, our heart leaps. The sense of awe and wonder we get when in nature comes from the heart. Of course, like any other attribute it can be unbalanced. Gold faucets are repulsive when there are so many in the world without.

Natural beauty is healing and connects us to life and spirit. As we saw in chapter 2, we are intimately connected to nature by means of the five natural elements in our bodies and our psyches. When in nature we feel this synergy and, if we listen closely, we can even hear spiritual messages.

Energy for Life

To find our way forward in life we must follow our hearts. This has been said countless times at high school and college graduations. However, having a want without the energy to back it up doesn't work.

Like the dementors in the Harry Potter stories, samskaras here suck the life energy out and one can feel fatigue and inertia. Wanting many things but without the ability to put forth the energy to get it. John frequently talked about how hard everything is. We followed this dynamic to the heart chakra and Traya revealed:

> …*After my parents divorced when I was twelve, I was engaged in a constant effort to get anything I needed. I would ask my mother for new shoes and I would get, "Get your father to buy them for you." I would ask my father and he would say, "Get it from your mother. I gave her money."*
>
> …*I would get angry and yell at them and I became an angry kid, and that is the only thing that gave me energy to go on. It pulled me out of my inertia temporarily.*

When working with the heart chakra, one will come to a layer of anger. The heart is angry for not getting what it needs. This anger too must be healed. It usually comes up near the end of the heart chakra healing process because the mind, as noted by John, needs the anger energy to counter the sad inertia energy that comes from suppressed life energy in the heart.

Knowledge

The heart chakra is in the realm of spirit, and truth comes to us not as intellectual understanding but as a knowing. "I know in my heart that it is true." This resonance with truth cannot come from the solar plexus chakra because it is time-bound and limited, and truth is timeless and limitless. The heart guides us away from that which is not good for us and toward that which is good. If we are connected to self we always know when we are heading in the wrong direction because the heart signals us by contracting and/or a sudden feeling of emptiness. (See chapter 5 for a discussion of the inner compass of which the heart chakra is a key component.)

Sara has been working on taking down her "defenses" while healing the solar plexus chakra and is now more aware of her lack of connection to herself and others. Now we approach the heart chakra by exploring her disconnection energy:

> ...It feels like I have no heart to connect with or stay true to.

Thus, she cannot trust the intuitive knowledge in her heart yet.

Hope, Motivation, Enthusiasm, and Joie de Vivre

One of my Muslim clients, while working with a samskaric heart chakra, said:

> ...There is a saying in Islam that if you lose hope, you don't believe in God.

This is an interesting viewpoint affirming that both a connection to spirit and a connection to hope abide in the heart. In order to be motivated, you must have hope. Hope is life affirming. Muriel was struggling with hopelessness energy and maintained that she didn't want to be hopeful because then she would be again subject to disappointment. I encouraged her by pointing out that if her fear energy can be healed (which we did by working with the solar plexus chakra) then her hopelessness can also be healed. She wasn't having any of it because she maintained:

....All the reading, talking, and studying positive thinking I did over the years—affirmations are crap!

It is important, when working with "down energy," to just keep going and not give in to the negativity that comes up. At some point it is going to switch to positive, uplifting energy and we just have to hang in there until it does. It is not like the solar plexus chakra where the fear keeps going down, down, down as you work with it. With the heart, as this down energy is surfaced, you are connecting more to yourself and, therefore, to the negative energy in the heart chakra and it will dominate the mind whenever you hook into it. When working with down energy it is helpful, in between Traya sessions, to disengage by focusing the attention at the pelvic chakra and repeat its bija vam as you would a mantra. This will help to keep the mind engaged there and its energy will dominate the mind and the "down" energy in the heart chakra will recede. Even though the negativity in the heart chakra is decreasing every time you work with it, it doesn't always feel that way—until it does and the positive aspects of the heart chakra bloom, particularly hope, motivation, enthusiasm, and joie de vivre.

Spirit versus Religion

Whenever we see others as different or less than, we are projecting an unhealthy heart chakra. The religions of the world were begun to bring people closer to spirit but, being a solar plexus chakra construct (trying to impose structure on spirituality), they have the opposite effect and actually separate groups of people. Remember, the heart chakra provides a sense of connection to self, others, nature, and spirit.

Religious divisions play out in the heart. These wider patterns of grouping around religion or ethnicity impact all of us individually. This "separation energy" produces samskaras in all of our hearts as we all must live in this world. I recently saw a quote by Deepak Chopra that counters this separating energy: "Jesus wasn't a Christian, Buddha wasn't a Buddhist, and Mohammed wasn't a Mohammedan."[14]

Spiritual practice encourages us to escape our judgments, grasping, and striving and live instead from our hearts. That is our true heart's desire: to put down petty desires for material things and live from the pure desire of our heart for connection with self. When we are connected to self, we are connected to everyone and everything, we understand truth and a real spiritual awakening happens.

Diamond Heart Chakra (Vajrahridaya)

• **Location:** at the sternum between the breasts

• **Function:** self-esteem

Vajrahridaya lies at the sternum between the solar plexus I-consciousness and the heart's connection consciousness and governs self-esteem. I call this secondary chakra "Diamond Heart," because when it is healthy, there is a sense of unbreakable strength—the opposite of the profound vulnerability which abides there when it is samskaric. When you think of the self-esteem chakra, think of feeling important to others. The feeling that abides here when samskaric is especially painful. This is, perhaps, the most vulnerable spot in the human psyche. For example, imagine that you are a child and go with your family to an extended family holiday party. All of the many children there have nice presents waiting for them—except for you! Imagine how that would feel. This is the feeling that one carries when this chakra is samskaric. Why not me? Feeling undeserving, it becomes difficult to seize opportunities and get one's due in life. It makes you want to hang back. "Do I really want to be out there?" One is too willing to accept scraps without understanding why or even questioning why. So this small but key chakra has a major impact on how we live our lives and achieve our dreams or not. The following are examples of the types of experiences that diminish self-esteem energy.

14. Deepak Chopra, "Powell's Book Interview with Dave Welch," *West By Northwest*, Marchq , 2001, http://www.westbynorthwest.org/springlate01/deepak/index. shtml.

Donna grew up with a chronically sick mother and an emotionally absent father:

…Feeling ignored made me feel unworthy.

Gloria was bullied as a child and in several emotionally abusive romantic relationships:

…My heart is bleeding from the inside. Low self-esteem prevents you from being able to defend yourself.
…What I went through wasn't important to others. They ignored it and asked me to ignore it too.

Sara has been hard at the Traya work, sees many changes, and is now focused on bringing the right relationship into her life. The following came up:

…I am taking good care of myself now and I will be a super healthy person that no one wants to be around. I am only setting myself up to enjoy being alone a bit more.

We then traced this belief to:

…When I was a teenager, everything seemed to be going fine. I had a boyfriend and both of us were interested and then suddenly it was done. No explanation. He drifted away and slept with my friend. They don't find enough in me to remain interested.
…I am a friendly, helpful person. Helpful substitutes for being wanted. Oh, I know where you can get one of those or you can borrow mine. It doesn't help. I have no other currency—I am not funny, interesting, or attractive.
…I was sprayed with Eau de Unlovable. I felt dismissed by everyone around me.

Her adoption experience—the original wound to her self-esteem —set her up to feel unwanted, unimportant (to her original parents), and uninteresting. Then other experiences were layered on that, reinforcing her sense of being unlovable and unimportant to others.

Sheryl was having difficulties in her relationship with her adult son.

...Mother used to badmouth me to other people. I was the only one of the children she did that to and my brother told me later how it upset him to hear it. I feel like my son is doing the same to me.

...I didn't think I was important enough to feel my mother shouldn't do it.

Carolyn was having trouble finding direction career-wise:

...It felt like other kids in school had normal homes and families but not me. So everything was for everyone else but me.

...In searching for a job the feeling is that there is nothing (that I would want) out there for me.

If you believe that having a job that aligns with your talents and interests is for others, then the likelihood of finding it is remote if not impossible.

Lorna, who is working to heal her fears and the idea that "I can't trust that everything will come out OK," was led to the self-esteem chakra in one of our sessions:

...My friend was over and hit her head on the swing set. My mother blamed me. With my mother you didn't protest. My point of view was not important.

Gloria is struggling in a job where she can't do the things that she loves. She has started writing for an online mystery magazine but sometimes doesn't keep up with it. Working here regarding this procrastination, she said:

...My needs were trampled on. Now I need to value what is important to me.

Indeed, it was a great joy for me to discover the self-esteem chakra with its ability to reverse the low self-esteem that I still carried around despite years of spiritual practice.

••• EXERCISE: TRAYA PRACTICE AT THE ••• HEART CHAKRA (ANAHATA)

Grounding

Ground by sitting up straight, focusing on the soles of your feet, and breathing in and out of the soles of your feet.

Use of Technique

Remember the thoughts that you identified in the chapter 1 exercise (Observing the Pain Body) and use one of them or use the basic technique in which you focus on a chakra and ask, "What memories are here?"

> **Step 1: Focus**—Keep your attention on the heart chakra in the center of the chest and breathe in and out gently.
>
> **Step 2: Surface**—Adopt the letting stance and ask, "What memories are here?"
>
> **Step 3: Release**—Note the memory and start to let negative energy go out by visualizing it coming out of the chakra. Go back to step 2 and surface another memory. You are continuously adding to the outflow of negative energy memory by memory. After you are finished surfacing memories for this session, let all of the negative energy go out and wait until the outflow stops.
>
> **Step 4: Replace and Imprint**—Visualize positive energy coming in (rays from the sun) and taking up the space that was taken up by the negative energy that went out. Ask, "What is this positive energy bringing in with it?" Note the words that appear in your mind.
>
> **Step 5: Scene from Nature (Optional)**—Breathe in and out while focusing attention on the heart chakra and let a scene from nature

appear in your mind. Note if the air (oxygen) energy element is strong. (See the list of chakra elements in chapter 2.)

It is always good to ground yourself in your body by again focusing on the soles of your feet and gently breathing in and out, especially after working with the higher chakras.

••• EXERCISE: TRAYA PRACTICE AT THE ••• SELF-ESTEEM CHAKRA (VAJRAHRIDAYA)

Let's use the manifestation technique this time. You are aware that your self-esteem can use some improvement. You look on the chart and locate self-esteem at vajrahridaya. Then continue with the Traya practice. You ground by breathing in and out of the soles of your feet.

Step 1: Focus—Keep your attention at the sternum and breathe in and out gently.

Step 2: Surface—Adopt the letting stance and ask, "What memories are here?"

Step 3: Release—Note the memory and start to let negative energy go out by visualizing it coming out of the chakra. Then either go back to step 2 and surface another memory and then repeat step 3 or proceed to step 4. Keep surfacing memories and adding to the chain of negative energy going out.

Step 4: Replace and Imprint—Visualize positive energy coming in (rays from the sun) and taking up the space that was taken up by the negative energy that went out. Ask, "What is this positive energy bringing in with it?" Note the words that appear in your mind.

There is no scene from nature step with the secondary chakras. Finish by grounding.

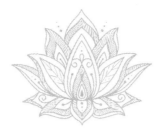

Chapter 10

THE THROAT CHAKRA (VISHUDDHA) AND THE TRUE SPEECH (SATYAVADYA) AND ASKING (SATYAHRIDAYA) CHAKRAS

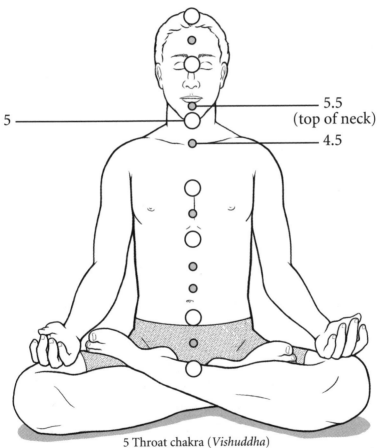

5 Throat chakra (*Vishuddha*)
5.5 True speech chakra (*Satyavadya*)
4.5 Asking chakra (*Satyahridaya*)

Figure 10: Fifth Chakra

Vishuddha, the Throat Chakra

- **Function:** self-expression
- **Attributes:** communication, identity, organization, authenticity, spontaneity, extroversion, wisdom, impact, leadership, space, expressiveness, listening, visibility
- **Attribute paradox:** "I talk a lot because I don't feel heard and then am not heard because I talk a lot."
- **Common issues in vishuddha:** hard to take up vocal space, being seen or heard, poor self-image

The throat chakra is still within the realm of elements and its element is ether. The Indian philosophers taught that ether has sound for its quality.[15] If we imagine that the physical elements came into being in the direction of subtlest to most dense, first would be ether, then air, then fire, then water, then earth. We could say that the rest of the elements came out of the ether. This is in accord with yogic teachings in which sound is thought to be the original element and the other four arise from it.

All cultures recognize the power of sound and have chants, prayers, magic incantations and mantras to influence both the inner and outer worlds. The Sanskrit term *mantra* is defined as a mystical verse or charm. As we saw in chapter 2, Sanskrit mantras activate the chakras and stimulate latent spiritual energy.

While it is true that sound is produced by the vocal cords in the physical body and not by the throat chakra itself, it influences the quality of sound and its effectiveness. All of the chakras transfer energy, but the throat chakra is unique in that it makes possible the production of physical sound waves that travel through the ether and are picked up by others. Sound has impact. Indeed, the term that best imparts the function of the throat chakra is "impact." Words are powerful and we create our world with words. We can make someone happy with our words or we can hurt them. It is with our words that we con-

---

15. George Feuerstein, *The Yoga Tradition: Its History, Literature, Philosophy and Practice* (Prescott, AZ: Holm Press, 2001), 201.

vey knowledge and information, entertain, converse, and influence others. We allow others to see us by revealing our thoughts and feelings. Our manner of speech provides information as to our identity. Whenever we speak we are exposed.

People with healthy throat chakra energy express themselves clearly and effectively *and* are heard. They act and speak spontaneously and authentically, fully expecting and receiving positive feedback and results. Engaged with others and in life, they organize their environment and life so as to achieve maximum effectiveness. Their work reflects their core values, beliefs, and purpose in life. Their words influence and inspire others. Their ability to listen and speak is well balanced and they are guided by their inner voice. They select their words carefully and do not speak ill of others. In summary, it is the opposite of hiding. It is the self on display without holding back—showing our full colors like the peacock.

Samskaras here cause us to feel unsafe expressing ourselves and to hold back from participating fully. The following client examples illustrate some of the many different ways samskaras can affect the throat chakra and prevent it from functioning fully.

Identity

Our ID cards show our picture, name, and date of birth. A "higher" chakra, the throat chakra moves us to ask the questions, "Who am I really? Am I this body, this personality, these desires, thoughts, feelings, and beliefs? What is my true identity?" As we heal the throat chakra, we prepare ourselves for work with the third eye (ajna) and the crown (sahasrara) chakras and the spiritual truths they reveal, including our true identity. In healing the throat chakra, we examine how we are functioning in life and if we are living in alignment with our purpose.

Our feelings, attitudes, beliefs, and values are displayed by our facial expressions, body language, how we dress, and especially our speech. What we show to the world, however, does not always reflect how we see ourselves from deep within. As we grow and mature, our self-image is influenced by how others respond to us. Negative input from others can have a crippling effect, causing us to shrink from people and life.

Working with the throat chakra will turn around a negative self-image. Brian saw himself as a failure, and his life reflected this idea. He lived this reality by working in a field he wasn't prepared or suitable for and being unsuccessful. He blamed himself for never applying himself in school. After working with the throat chakra (and other chakras), he went back to school and became an excellent pupil, speaking out in class and receiving accolades from his teachers and other students. "I never thought I would hear so many good things being said about me. I am no longer a failure—I am a winner." Brian changed his self-image by healing the throat chakra and then living more authentically, studying for work that was more closely aligned with who he is.

Summer, a sales coach working with groups in seminars, complains how teaching "takes so much out of me. I push through when teaching, but I am never comfortable." When we explored the throat chakra, we found she had the unconscious belief:

…No one wants to hear from me. I am nobody. I don't exist.

This memory came up:

…My parents talked over me. They never listened.

Rationally, she knows that her audience wants and needs to hear from her, but these unconscious beliefs contribute to her struggle to teach even though she is good at it.

Spontaneity

When we act spontaneously, we act from what is coming up naturally within us. Indeed, it is our enthusiasm for particular activities that help us find our path in life. The buoyant energy of the playful kitten, pup, or child seems to just bubble up and spill over without restriction. As we mature, this energy naturally balances but will become restricted if we experience negative feedback from others when acting spontaneously. A memory from Evelyn's childhood in Taiwan that came to her when she was working with the throat chakra illustrates this point:

> ... When I was eight, I was living in the country with my grandmother and went home with a new friend after school through the countryside. I didn't realize how far it was and that I would not be able to get back home that same night. There were no telephones, so I couldn't contact my grandmother. When we arrived at school the next morning, the entire school was waiting. The principal put us on the stage in front of everyone and told everyone not to be like us. We were embarrassed.

Then there is the type of spontaneity related to speaking up in challenging moments. Katarina sometimes feels browbeaten at work by her boss, who is asking her why she is not able to keep up with the work. In reality she is often interrupted by demanding people from other departments and is unable to keep them at bay, taking time from her work. She is unable to respond to her boss truthfully and let him know it is the constant interruptions that affect her performance. Katarina often thinks of what she will say in anticipation of a stressful situation or what she should have said after the situation but in the moment becomes mute. We explored the throat chakra and the following samskaric memories surfaced:

> ... In middle school I was teased mercilessly, and when I tried to defend myself, it only made it worse. They took my words and used them against me.

A charismatic authority figure in an organization she belonged to questioned her about one of her decisions:

> ... He was like a cult leader. He always finds the way to win the argument and you are always wrong.

A former roommate had a forceful and domineering personality:

> ... You can't win an argument or make a point. Everything you say is wrong.

Even though she has a good point to make with the boss and if she speaks up it may impact her job positively, she is conditioned not to defend herself. These negative communication experiences began with the middle school experiences that then generated the negative tendency (vasana) of not speaking up while, at the same time, attracting situations that challenge her to do so. After clearing these "not speaking up" samskaras, she not only spoke up for herself but convinced her boss to move her into a better job.

Communication and Authenticity

The throat chakra is closely related to the pelvic chakra—the "relationship" chakra. They both deal with space in relation to others. With the pelvic chakra, the emphasis is on physical and emotional space and with the throat chakra the emphasis is on vocal space. The throat chakra is also a relationship chakra because when we communicate it is with another person. Communication allows us to connect with others, solidify relationships, show who we are, share ideas and information, and diminish negative emotions. We all know that when we are upset or confused, talking to someone with a sympathetic ear helps.

As we saw in chapter 1, everything, including thoughts, is composed of energy. Disturbing thoughts have uncomfortable energy because they are foreign to our innate positive psychic energy structure. Talking about them with someone releases some of this energy, and the mind can shift. Though the samskaras remain, they may become less active for a period of time. This phenomenon of energy releasing when we talk about something can also happen when we don't want it to. For example, if we talk too much about a creative project we are considering or involved in, some energy may leak and cause us to lose interest in the project or become distracted by something else and shift our focus entirely. This is why writers often will not talk about their work before it is finished.

It is important for us to communicate well with everyone, but especially with those closest to us. This energy was out of balance in Lotus's home:

…My parents were either not speaking or exploding.

The following case highlights the importance of clear communication in relationships.

Sheryl is an older woman who is young in spirit and leads an active life including heading up her own business. She is generally talkative, but I noticed that there was something off about her communication. She frequently did not provide sufficient information and would become annoyed when I asked for clarification. Despite my highlighting this communication pattern, she was unable to change it until we removed the related samskaras from the throat chakra. We were working on her relationship with her adult son who kept her at "arm's length." She felt she had to "tiptoe" around him so he wouldn't lash out. Traya revealed the following:

…I am not able to speak because he doesn't want to hear from me.

She is referring to the current situation with her son. I ask, "What memories are here related to not being able to speak?" Immediately, she remembers her mother yelling at her:

…My parents didn't see me as a human being, just a child servant. They didn't want to hear from me.
…The family dynamic was that we never talked about what was going on. I was never permitted to speak out.
…I had to turn myself inside out to avoid trouble and now I am being asked to adjust myself for my son's comfort.

This last memory points directly to the function of the throat chakra—can I be authentic or do I have to "adjust myself" for other people's comfort? Three weeks later they had a forty-five minute spontaneous conversation "out of the blue." Sheryl felt that for the first time, they were each able to be truthful with each other. Her son confided some family dynamics that Sheryl was unaware of and this confidence brought them closer. The "arm's length" energy had shifted. When energy shifts, even in only one of the people in a relationship, things change.

Extroversion/Visibility

I think of this chakra as peacock energy. The peacock is the consummate extrovert. The throat chakra is extroversion energy in the sense of no holding back, spontaneity, and no hiding out—feeling safe enough to be truly yourself and take up verbal space. A saying that Evelyn heard often in her childhood in China came up as a samskara when she was working with the throat chakra:

> *…Be like the wheat; when it is fully grown, it bows down.*

The wheat seeds filling the plant weigh it down and the entire field looks like bowing wheat. This essentially means that if you are successful, you should be humble. This contrasts with the peacock energy as the wheat proverb message is "don't stand out." Essentially, the throat chakra energy is about coming out of hiding and being seen. Like the roaring lion, we feel completely safe in being seen and in expressing ourselves. The lion isn't boasting; he is being himself.

Hiding is often obvious. Typically someone may be shy, have difficulty interacting with others, and live with some degree of isolation. This was true of Zoe, who feels uncomfortable around people and has difficulty contributing to group conversations. She revealed the following during Traya:

> *…I was once called out by my friend in front of others for not knowing what I was talking about.*
> *…Feeling on the spot in class or people disliking what I am trying to contribute—people would get frustrated with me when sharing in class.*

But sometimes hiding is not so obvious and can actually look like the opposite. People can hide behind talking. Remember that a chakra can be out of balance by being overactive as well as being underactive. When you are not speaking up, it may appear to others that this energy is weak, and when you speak too much it can look like the energy is very strong. We all know what it is like to spend time with someone who doesn't listen and talks about themselves incessantly. This may look like extroversion, but in fact they are hiding behind their words. It is a "word wall" and we feel shut out, get bored, and tune out. Effective communication includes listening. A healthy throat chakra balances speaking and listening, allowing for true interaction.

It is important not only to be seen but to be seen in the right way. The following memory came up for Francine while working at the throat:

> ...I was always an excellent athlete and enjoyed competitions. I realized as a young teenager that I was being looked at but not seen. Men were ogling me and it felt very uncomfortable. I quit.

Masks and False Personas

At the beginning of our session, Lisa states, "I am so tired of pretending with my boss. I have to be pleasant when I hate my job and don't value the things that she values. I want to live more authentically." Traya led us to the throat chakra:

> ...I smiled hoping that Mommy and Daddy, who were miserable, would be happy.
> ...In my waitress job I always had to be "on," smiling and being pleasant, when that is not how I felt.

Tamara presented an upbeat exterior. During Traya work, she became aware that she picked this up from her mother:

> ...Mom was always happy on the surface. She laughed too loud and too hard. It was so irritating—she was always "on." My brother, when little, asked her to stop smiling so much.
> ...I can't have a conversation with my mother. She always falls back on anecdotes. She is not capable of a give-and-take conversation.

Communication and Skillful Speech

What we say is just as important as how much we say. When this chakra is healthy, speaking and listening are balanced and we speak skillfully.

Brian wants desperately to "have a voice," yet finds that he still operates from a defensive position and this interferes with his communication. His wife was visiting family in Florida and she called him to tell him that two people in the room were having birthdays and he should wish them a happy birthday. At the moment she reached him, he was finishing up some work and was expecting a visitor. Instead of saying, "this is a bad time" and "I will call back" or briefly wishing them happy birthday and getting right off of the phone, he became defensive and with annoyance, saying, "I am busy." When his wife returned home, she angrily accused him of not caring about her family. Traya revealed:

> …My father was always lecturing me—talking at me.

His wife hadn't asked him if it was a good time to speak.

> …He was like a dragon spitting fire at me and I feel a low-level anxiety—waiting for someone to impose something on me.
> …I feel as though everyone is trying to strangle me.
> …With my father everything was a fait accompli—no one had any voice in decisions. With my wife I often feel it is "my way or the highway."

This clearly shows why he couldn't perceive the correct action or words in the situation—he was feeling and acting (reacting) as though his wife was imposing something on him instead of thoughtfully trying to include him. This is a good example of how samskaras interfere with skillful communication.

The Buddha outlined the Noble Eightfold Path to freedom from suffering. Right Speech is one of these eight suggested precepts. In the Abhaya Sutra, in which the Buddha is responding to questions from Prince Abhaya, we see that Right Speech is that which is true, beneficial, and timely.[16] Essentially, something that is untrue is not said and something that is true but not beneficial is not said. Something that is true and beneficial is only said at the right time. This is Right Speech. Indeed, the Buddha was skillful with speech, using the right words with the right audience according to their capacity to understand.

---

16. Thanssaro Bhikkhu, trans. *Abhaya Raja Kumara Sutta*, http://buddhasutra.com/files/Buddhist_Sutra_A1.pdf, accessed January 2017, 34.

Bad speech can also hurt the speaker. When you cause suffering in the world with bad speech, you cannot be free from the suffering that you are creating because you are putting it out into the world in which you live. Brian's unskillful speech demonstrates this. His wife became angry and then came home and confronted him. Now they are both suffering.

The throat chakra enables skillful and correct speech. This is a powerful energy and we must use it wisely and consciously. Just as great harm can be done with incorrect speech, a lot of good can be done with correct speech. We have seen how the voice of one person such as the Buddha can influence so many and change the world for the better. *Ahimsa*, or "nonharming," provides a foundation for the skillful use of this energy through which we can express love from the heart chakra located below the throat chakra, along with the intuitive wisdom of the third eye chakra, which lies above.

Organization, Leadership, and Impact

Brian struggles with organization. We saw earlier that he had many issues at the throat chakra as a result of his father talking at and over him. He also grew up in a chaotic and disorganized household. When he went back to school, he was worried that he would be unsuccessful partly because of his "failure" identity but also because of his poor organizational skills. He knew that one of the reasons he had done poorly in college the first time around was his failure to allow the appropriate amount of time for each assignment. With our focus on healing the throat chakra, Brian was able to ace all of his classes and surprised himself by actually being ahead of everyone else with projects and being the one whom the other students came to with questions about material covered in class, upcoming assignments, and deadlines.

Why is organization an attribute of the throat chakra, which is functionally the self-expression chakra? In order to use language well you must organize your words, sentences, and thoughts. You can't have language without organization. Organization creates efficiency and efficiency supports accomplishment. When you organize, you open up space for ideas to flow and plans to form that outline actions to be taken. When this energy is healthy, you are able to open up space in your life for the things that are most important to you.

We saw that one of the important attributes of the throat chakra is impact. In order to have an impact, ideas must be coherently organized, presented, and implemented. When we are well organized, have good ideas, and can communicate well, people often look to us for leadership.

Creative Expression

We all have something unique to communicate. We have to not only find our voice and heal our fear of using our voice, but we must feel we have something to say and that others want to hear what we have to express. While we were working with the throat chakra, Sara said:

> …What good is it to be more articulate if I have nothing to say that anyone wants to hear?

The impact of negative energy in the throat chakra reminds me of the hungry ghosts of Buddhism. These metaphorical beings live in the hungry ghost realm with big empty stomachs and mouths so tiny and necks so long and thin they cannot swallow anything so they are always desperately hungry. They represent the afflictive state of a greedy mind trying desperately to take in but be never satisfied. With a blocked throat chakra, we may have more difficulty in both sending energy out (speaking) and taking things in (listening). Desperately hungry for expression, our mouths and ears won't open because of the false beliefs created by samskaras such as with Sara from earlier:

> …I don't have anything worthwhile to say.

Speaking with his writing teacher, Brian said, "I am starting to wonder if what I am saying is worth saying."

The teacher responded, "If you think it is, it is."

Later on in our work, I heard his growth and self-confidence come through when he said, "I am a writer because I say so. It has taken me years to be able to say that."

Inner Voice, Wisdom, and Dreams

When you believe that what you say matters, then what comes from your inner voice matters too and wisdom appears. When this energy is healthy, the inner voice comes through loud and clear.

Dreams are messages from the deep mind organized and communicated through this chakra. Dreams are ethereal (the throat chakra is the ether element) and often difficult to remember. Unless you write it down right away, you will forget it unless it is very dramatic. If you forget parts of the dream, focus at the throat chakra similar to the Traya focus technique and ask to remember more of the dream. Often it will come back to you.

Space and Expression

Taking up vocal space involves self-expression, spontaneity, and assertiveness. To have a voice means to be the principal in your own life. This is a particularly significant issue for women. Studies show that women who speak up in the business world are not taken as seriously or viewed as favorably as men doing the exact same thing. This example comes from the *New York Times*:

> YEARS ago, while producing the hit TV series "The Shield," Glen Mazzara noticed that two young female writers were quiet during story meetings. He pulled them aside and encouraged them to speak up more.
>
> Watch what happens when we do, they replied.
>
> Almost every time they started to speak, they were interrupted or shot down before finishing their pitch. When one had a good idea, a male writer would jump in and run with it before she could complete her thought.
>
> Sadly, their experience is not unusual.
>
> We've both seen it happen again and again. When a woman speaks in a professional setting, she walks a tightrope. Either she's barely heard or she's judged as too aggressive. When a

man says virtually the same thing, heads nod in appreciation for his fine idea. As a result, women often decide that saying less is more.[17]

It is especially important for women to heal the throat chakra in order to speak freely and be heard and taken seriously. Most likely each of these women in this article has "not being heard" samskaras in the throat chakra and that too contributes to the male behavior. When they are removed, that will also influence the male behavior for the better, for their communication energy will be more powerful and they will make themselves heard without effort—or calling it out when it doesn't happen in a skillful way. Remember that healthy communication energy involves speaking, listening, *and* being heard. So if the throat chakra is healthy, all three of those are more likely to appear at the same time, regardless of the audience.

Vocal space energy also means to allow space in our life for our path to appear so that we may express our full potential. Sometimes this involves allowing silence in. Remember, we can hide behind too many words also. There are times when nothing need be said and we need to be comfortable with that too.

Asking Chakra (Satyahridaya)

- **Location:** top of the chest near depression between the collarbones, between the heart chakra (anahata) and the throat chakra (vishuddha)
- **Function:** to ask for what is in the heart

This chakra lies between the heart chakra and the throat chakra and, as with all secondary chakras, contains qualities of each of its neighboring primary chakras—the heart where we are true to ourselves, and the throat's self-expression energy. Therefore, *satyahridaya*'s function is asking for what is in the heart—for what we truly

---

17. Sheryl Sandberg and Adam Grant, "Speaking While Female: Why Women Stay Quiet at Work," *The New York Times* Sunday Review, January 12, 2015, SR3.

want. *Hridaya* is Sanskrit for "heart" and *satya* means "truth." (Therefore: "truth-heart.")

Sheila was led to this area in one of our sessions. When we focused here, the following came to her mind:

> ...I see myself as a child being swept along by my parents and older siblings. I was just moved from one place to another and had no say in anything. I could never ask for what I wanted because I was so disconnected from myself due to the lack of attention that I didn't know what I wanted. Or even that I had a right to want anything. I was like a barnacle attached to the family organism just going along without a say in anything.

Not only did she have difficulty expressing her needs to significant others but she couldn't allow herself to express a desire for a better life—for work that was more in line with who she is and for better relationships.

Sara told me, "Nothing stirs me." This led us to the asking chakra and the following:

> ...What comes out serves "Let's not have a conflict" rather than "no." My words are a traitor to my heart. For example, I didn't tell a guy that I was dating that it was not working even though I felt that way.

Further exploration led us to the experience(s) that made her feel that she couldn't express what was in her heart:

> ...When I was eight, my sister was seven. She was difficult and distant and my parents went to greater lengths to get her to connect. My mom taught her how to sew. I remember asking Mom, "Can we do something just you and me?" Nothing happened. I asked for something that I clearly wanted and nothing happened. So I felt that I was trespassing by asking and that I didn't deserve the attention that wasn't mine.

True Speech Chakra (Satyavadya)

- **Location:** between the throat chakra (vishuddha) and the third eye chakra (ajna), at the top of the neck at the crease where the neck meets the head
- **Function:** true speech

Just what is truth? Zen teaches that truth is what is happening right now in this moment. Experience is truth rather than opinions, ideas, and beliefs. If I tell you that a tea I am pouring in your cup has a delicate floral and nutty taste, this is my opinion. The taste of the tea at the moment you experience it is your truth.

Satyavadya (true speech) is another secondary chakra lying between two primary chakras. As such, it has aspects of the throat chakra below and the third-eye chakra above. In the third eye chakra we see the truth and in the throat chakra hear, speak, and live truth.

The following element from a Traya session with Sheryl is revealing of the function of this chakra. Though she had no awareness of this before our session, I feel it imparts an important truth for her and for our society as a whole:

> *…I remember elementary school. I came from a dysfunctional and neglectful home and I felt very lost. I felt neglected in school also. I never said anything about what I was feeling because I knew they weren't interested. There was only one purpose in being there— for me to take in their information, not for me to speak my truth.*

In our educational systems, we shove information down the students' throats, so to speak, but rarely try to find out who they are and what their life is like. Just come, sit in the chair, listen to *us*, and repeat it back to us. School represents the outside world to these kids and the message is "You are not important; only what we have to teach you is important."

We can see how the Traya process itself is healing for her because now we are paying attention to her truth. When you are cut off from your truth, you are cut off from your power. When you are in your truth, you don't doubt yourself.

The throat chakra and its two associated secondary chakras, the asking chakra and the true speech chakra, help us to express our voice in the world so we can bloom fully and make a difference. When the throat chakra is healthy, the tendency is to speak out rather than hold back. Be sure to always work with lower chakras that are particularly out of balance (see scene from nature list in chapter 2), especially the pelvic chakra and solar plexus, before the throat chakra. Misperceptions and misunderstandings from samskaras in the lower chakras may "spill out" through the throat chakra if not addressed first. For example, if there is a lot of anger in the pelvic chakra or annoyance in the solar plexus chakra, you don't want to be constantly expressing it. That doesn't mean that you should not work with the throat chakra at all. It just means that you don't want to focus exclusively here and make a major change in the energy before there are positive resources available from healthier lower chakras. If you do work there, it is a good idea to start with listening skills.

••• EXERCISE: TRAYA PRACTICE AT THE ••• THROAT CHAKRA (VISHUDDHA)

Grounding
Ground by sitting up straight, focusing on the soles of your feet, and breathing in and out of the chakras at the soles of your feet.

Following Dreams Technique
This is another deep mind–guided technique. Dreams come through the throat chakra but can be pointing to the need to work in any chakra. You remember the dream and, while focusing on the body, then ask, "Where in me is the energy that this dream wants to surface?" You feel a strong sensation at the throat chakra. You then continue with the Traya steps while focusing here.

Step 1: Focus—Keep your attention on the throat chakra at the center of your neck and breathe in and out gently.

Step 2: Surface—Adopt the letting stance and ask, "What memories are here that this dream wants to surface."

Step 3: Release—Note the memory and start to let negative energy go out by visualizing it coming out of the chakra. After you begin the release process with this memory you can then ask, "What other memories are here?" Continuously add to the outflow of negative energy memory by memory. After you are finished surfacing memories for this session, let all of the negative energy go out and wait until the outflow stops.

Step 4: Replace and Imprint—Visualize positive energy coming in (rays from the sun) and taking up the space that was taken up by the negative energy that went out. Ask, "What is this positive energy bringing in with it?" Note the words that appear in your mind.

Step 5: Scene from Nature (Optional)—Breathe in and out while focusing attention on the throat chakra and let a scene from nature appear in your mind. Note if the ether (sky) element is strong. (See the scene from nature list in chapter 2.)

It is always good to ground yourself in your body by again focusing on the soles of your feet and gently breathing in and out, especially after working with the "higher" chakras.

••• EXERCISE: TRAYA PRACTICE AT THE •••
ASKING CHAKRA (SATYAHRIDAYA)

You use the following memories technique from chapter 8. As an example, you remember that you were afraid to ask for what you really wanted for your birthday because you feared you may not get it since your parents were arbitrary with presents. You are led to the asking chakra located near the depression in the center of the collarbone. Next is to continue with the Traya practice. You ground by breathing in and out of the soles of your feet.

Step 1: Focus—Keep your attention on the asking chakra and breathe in and out gently.

Step 2: Surface—You already have the memory so you don't need to surface it. After you begin the release process with this memory, you can then ask, "What other memories are here?"

Step 3: Release—Let the negative energy go out. When it stops proceed to step 4.

Step 4: Replace and Imprint—Visualize positive energy coming in (rays from the sun) and taking up the space that was taken up by the negative energy that went out. Ask, "What is this positive energy bringing in with it?" Note the words that appear in your mind.

There is no scene from nature step with the secondary chakras. Finish by grounding again.

••• EXERCISE: TRAYA PRACTICE AT THE ••• TRUE SPEECH CHAKRA (SATYAVADYA)

Use the following the body technique from chapter 7. Focus on your body and ask, "Where in me is there any energy that needs to surface?" You are led to the true speech chakra located at the top of the neck. Or you think of someone in your life whom you have difficulty speaking the truth to so you focus your attention here at the true speech chakra. Next is to continue with the Traya practice. You ground by breathing in and out of the soles of your feet.

Step 1: Focus—Keep your attention on the top of the neck and breathe in and out gently.

Step 2: Surface—Adopt the letting stance and ask, "What memories are here that are ready to come up to the surface?" After you begin the release process with this memory you can then ask, "What other memories are here?"

Step 3: Release—Let the negative energy go out. When it stops proceed to step 4.

Step 4: Replace and Imprint—Visualize positive energy coming in (rays from the sun) and taking up the space that was taken up by the negative energy that went out. Ask, "What is this positive energy bringing in with it?" Note the words that appear in your mind.

There is no scene from nature step with the secondary chakras. Finish by grounding again.

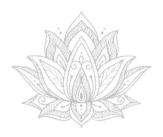

Chapter 11

THE THIRD EYE CHAKRA (AJNA)
AND THE INSIGHT CHAKRA (SATYAMANAS)

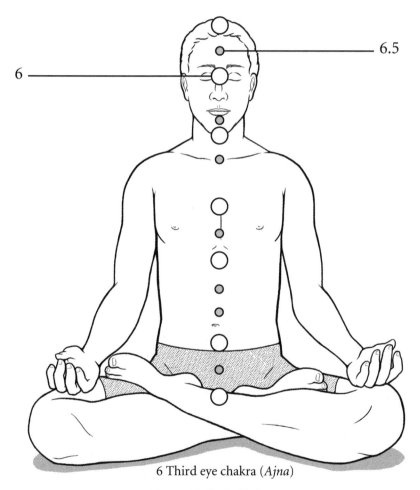

6 Third eye chakra (*Ajna*)

Figure 11: Sixth Chakra

Ajna, the Third Eye Chakra

- **Function:** clear perception
- **Attributes:** clarity, truth, timing, wide perspective, resolve, piercing illusions, intuition, vision, lucidity, acceptance, discernment, detachment, foresight, objectivity, wisdom
- **Attribute paradox:** "Truth is a matter of perception."
- **Common issues in ajna:** denial, lack of clarity or perception, discounts intuition

The third eye chakra and the crown chakra (sahasrara) connect to universal consciousness beyond the limitations of space and time. They operate on a higher plane beyond the five earthly elements of the lower five chakras.

Perceive Truth

The third eye chakra is perception without reason, complementing and balancing the solar plexus chakra's rational and logical tendencies. Often referred to as the "sixth sense," it expands our sensory field, enabling us to see the truth in any situation. If the elephant is standing in the middle of the room, it is clearly visible. One not only sees the elephant, but its size, color, smell, and everything else about the elephant. One also knows how the elephant got there and what purpose it is serving to be there. All of the information is taken in. The truth of the situation is perceived and accepted. The third eye chakra provides the ability to see beyond deceit and false personas.

You may not be able to explain rationally why you know but you do. Here we understand the difference between having an idea about something and being aware.

One also understands the implications of this clear perception. Unlike the solar plexus chakra's dualistic approach to understanding, the third eye chakra perceives truth without judgment.

When the third eye chakra is samskaric, one cannot see the truth even when they are hit over the head with it over and over again. Maybe one grew up in a confusing situation where obvious issues were not addressed and/or grew up surrounded by ugliness that one doesn't want to see. Samskaras then form in the third eye chakra and produce the opposite of clear sight—denial. This denial energy then impacts the ability to see people, situations, and correct decisions clearly. Once denial energy is established, we can get involved in unhealthy situations and have difficulty getting out of them.

Denial is also known as an ego defense in traditional psychology. We all have or have had some of this in our lives. Denying the truth of someone's behavior toward us that we will not allow ourselves to perceive or accept. We stay in denial because it means that we can hold on to something that we do not want to let go of or it protects us when we are too fragile to handle the truth. The "defense" of denial is very powerful and ubiquitous. This is one of the mechanisms that supports addictions of all types and keeps people in jobs and relationships that are not good for them. Regardless of the often painful consequences (attaching to someone who is unsuitable) or that which can even be dire and life threatening (addictions), we convince ourselves that there is no problem or we can manage it.

The third eye chakra helps guide one through the formative years while other aspects of the self are being developed. Those in situations of neglect or abuse and without guidance from adults lose this faculty due to a samskaric third eye chakra. The small child does not have the emotional resources or coping skills to handle the truth of dysfunctional experiences, especially when they feel powerless to do anything about it. Although the deep mind registers the truth, the third eye chakra keeps this understanding unconscious. Any powerfully dissonant experience impacts on many different levels at the same time. The third eye chakra becomes samskaric because the truth is too painful, the heart chakra becomes samskaric because the child feels abandoned and unloved, and the solar plexus chakra becomes samskaric because feelings must be held back in order to be in control.

Children who must live in denial to cope with their circumstances suffer particularly from poor choices and then blame themselves for these choices the rest of their lives. Myrna started using drugs and behaved promiscuously as a teenager. Now in her thirties, she still has flashbacks of some of the more humiliating things that she did, and she is having difficulty forgiving herself. She is beginning to understand that she did not have the guidance of her parents and her internal guidance system was not functioning either—few if any inner resources. She was acting out the low self-esteem and poor boundaries resulting from her familial dysfunction. She couldn't see that this was harmful to her at the time that she engaged in it. She was able to stop the drug use, finish school, and become successful in the publishing business, but she has difficulty giving herself credit for that. Which brings up another important fact—not only painful truths are blocked from consciousness but also positive truths. Once denial energy is established one cannot see or own the truth—good or bad. Denial is denial. She cannot see the truth that stopping the drug use and building a successful career against major odds was a significant accomplishment, nor does she give herself credit for her intelligence and talents. Dominating her mind are the negative samskaras and their associated thoughts and feelings related to her past behavior. The pain body is relentless.

One will often enter into jobs or careers because of denial about the prospects, the lack of fit, or the boring reality of the work. We can enter into and remain in abusive or otherwise unhealthy relationships because it is impossible to see the truth. Even if we can see it with the help of friends or professionals, we will continually slip back into denial.

One can even be in denial about the denial. Charles said to me, "I know that I am in denial, but I believe her anyway."

If there is a history of trauma, the third eye chakra should not be healed until the lower chakras are healthier—especially the solar plexus and the heart chakras—as an escape route should not be cut off until the need has been removed. Healthier lower chakras provide balance, strength, and inner resources that provide the ability to cope with unclouded reality.

Simon is involved in a difficult marriage with hostility often arising. He and his wife are also in couple's therapy with another therapist. He loves his wife and is confused about whether he should invest any more time into trying to heal the relationship or move on. Traya led us to the third eye chakra, from which the following memory arose:

> *...At around age ten, my mother took my cousin and me to Coney Island. When we came out of the subway, a man joined us. My mother acted as if we just ran into him, but it was clear to me that he was waiting for us. She introduced him as a coworker but I always suspected he was more than that because she was so interested in pleasing him. My cousin and I pretended that everything was OK but I was very uncomfortable. I never mentioned it to my father and never discussed it with anyone.*

When growing up we may become vaguely aware of situations or issues that are uncomfortable and "off." The people involved never speak about it or deal with it and the message is "better not go there." There is an unspoken agreement not to mention it. Simon perceived something "off" about this situation but put it out of his mind and went on with his life. The deep mind registers everything and a samskara formed in the third eye chakra so now he cannot see situations so clearly. He reverted to the solar plexus chakra: problem-solving, should I or shouldn't I, pros and cons. It is common that people don't know whether to rely on their intuition or their reason, as our society overvalues reason. The following quote acknowledges this flaw in our society:

> Albert Einstein called the intuitive or metaphoric mind a sacred gift. He added that the rational mind was a faithful servant. It is paradoxical that in the context of modern life we have begun to worship the servant and defile the divine.[18]

After working with the third eye chakra, Simon's perspective on the relationship changed from "Should I or should I not stay in the marriage?" to "Why am I allowing myself to live with so much anger? Why has it been acceptable for so long?" He was truly shocked that

---

18. Bob Samples, *The Metaphoric Mind: A Celebration of Creative Consciousness*, (Rolling Hills, CA: Jalmar Press, 1993), 19.

he had accepted the situation for so long. He then began to see how his behavior contributes to his wife's anger. It is indeed the truth that heals. We must see it before we can wholeheartedly confront a situation and resolve it. It was crucial for Simon to see that living with hostility is unacceptable in order to have his full voice in his couple's therapy and demand change while, at the same time, acknowledging that his behavior contributes to the hostility in the home.

When the third eye chakra is healthy, we can see our way to a better life.

Timelessness

In chapter 8, we saw that time is an illusion created by the solar plexus chakra's structure-creating attribute. The third eye chakra does not have that limitation and can perceive truth in the past, present, or future. As with other chakras, the third eye when samskaric can be either under or over active. When overactive, attributes of the third eye chakra will be exaggerated. For example, the solar plexus chakra's logical analytic aspects are exaggerated to excessive thinking and over-intellectualization or the throat chakra's self-expression function is exaggerated in excessive talking. With a significantly samskaric third eye chakra, one can develop an exaggerated ability to "see the future" or a psychic ability and can then become attached to it. There is a temptation to navigate through life in this way—always needing to know what is going to happen before it happens. This is an ineffective way to live, as overactive energy is not balanced or integrated with the other chakra energies. When the third eye chakra is strong, one no longer feels the need to consult seers. There is a general knowledge of the future, and one knows what decisions to make and paths to take without having to "tune in" to the future or consult psychics. This ability is one of the elements of our innate Inner Compass described in chapter 5.

Although the third eye chakra gives us a sense of the future, its main function is to give us a sense of the truth of our situation *now*, because our lives are not lived in the future but in the present. It is the decisions that we make now that affect our future. When information about the future comes through, it is so that you can do something now to avoid future difficulties. Future-focusing can be a trap. One can be so focused on the future that they forget that they need to take action now. When the chakras are balanced and integrated, one is not concerned about the details of the future because they are more grounded and involved in their life today and there is a sense of confidence and trust that everything will work out. When the third eye chakra is healthy, this "sixth sense" becomes like any other sense, an integrated part of our interaction with the everyday world. One can check in here when contemplating a decision or a new direction.

At times, the future will also come to you without looking for it. You will be thinking about something and then it will actually happen. This is precognition or extrasensory perception (ESP). Or your dreams will show you something about the future. A healthy third eye chakra is a powerful beacon that can always be depended on to show us the way.

Timing

Timing is everything. One knows not only what action to take but when to take it. This gives life the quality of going smoothly. I remember when I first realized how this worked. I had a job with lots of responsibility and many projects to move along. My desk had several piles of paper related to projects that needed to move. If I focused on the project that had the nearest deadline—the rational choice—I came up against various obstacles. Often I was unable to reach or get a response from key people. I soon realized that if I worked on the project that felt like it "had the most energy," it would move smoothly along. Answers would be readily available, necessary information would appear "out of the blue," and everyone was helpful. The third eye chakra was guiding me without my realizing it. I just "knew" which project to work on that day. We cannot make things happen according to our timetables. We can help things happen by trusting ourselves to know when to take action and when not to.

Detachment and Objectivity

One feels "above the fray" while remaining engaged and connected. New vistas open up and there is a sense of connection to a higher truth and detachment from ego. Detachment from ego is a healthy sense of the futility of ego-seeking behaviors. Knowing that trying to make things happen in this world rather than let them happen is ultimately futile. One also sees that it is futile to want or expect others to change.

When one can see the truth of a situation, one can be more objective and not personalizing or demonizing. This allows one to let go of attachment to resentments and past hurts. When one holds resentments, one is still attached energetically. Now, instead of resenting someone else's behavior, one can see "they didn't have what it took to provide me with what I needed," for example. One can see how others' suffering impedes them and not take things personally.

Elevation and Completeness

The third eye chakra provides a sense of being more than you thought because of a connection to a higher operative energy. It becomes clear that intuition is a spiritual force and there is a higher purpose underpinning our lives. Profound material often comes up when working with the third eye chakra.

In one session with Simon, the following came up:

> ...I'm in the country near woods as a kid. I remember feeling there has to be something more than what is seen. I have a heavy heart—there is something greater than I am and I am not connected to it.
> ...I remember our cat giving birth to kittens and felt the same way.
> ...The play of world pulls you in different directions and you lose sight of the bigger picture. It pops through, but then I am in denial it is really there.

Mark was raised in a structured religious denomination. He surfaced:

...I feel that religion is all just a bunch of fairy tales. I feel I am losing touch with spirit.

I asked him to keep the focus on the third eye chakra and ask, "What do I need to know?" The answer readily appeared:

...The origin of the universe begins with me. I must light my own way.

I also had a profound experience when working with the third eye chakra. I was removing samskaras and suddenly I saw the truth of who my parents actually were. They both appeared to me as they would have been as parents if they did not have so many wounds. They were both playful, attentive, accessible, and loving instead of removed, shut down, and inattentive. I saw the enormity of not only my loss, but also their samskaric imprisonment, and wept. The people I knew were like bizarre shadows of who they truly were, and I had never seen beyond these false personas. It reminded me of the scene in *Harry Potter and the Sorcerer's Stone* when he finally "meets" his parents as they were when he was a baby before they were killed. Now, I had already known all of this and had long ago forgiven my parents, but this was different—I saw clearly the reality of who they really were when unencumbered by samskaras and the truth of what all of us had missed out on. I chant for them now that they may have more of a full existence in their next lives. I am profoundly grateful for the Traya process that allows me to break the cycle of suffering and limitation and, unlike my parents, live a full life in this existence.

Stillness, Wisdom, and Resolve

Truth is unchanging and unmoving and has the essential characteristic of stillness. Wisdom comes from access to the truth. Wisdom allows one to know what, when, and how to respond to a difficult situation using skillful means. It is in stillness that one perceives and grows. Once this third eye chakra connection to wisdom happens, one no longer is attached to distractions but wants to be more present to more fully experience the higher self. Spiritual truths resonate and there are no doubts. There is a sense of certainty that what one perceives is the truth. This is the third eye chakra resolve.

Insight Chakra (Satyamanas)

• **Location:** center of forehead
• **Function:** insight

Satyamanas means "to turn the mind toward the truth." Lying between the third eye chakra's (ajna) seeing the truth and the crown chakra's (sahasrara) freedom, these functions are combined in profound insight. Insight is defined as "act or result of apprehending the inner nature of things or of seeing intuitively."[19] After thoroughly exploring an issue in the lower chakras—the insight chakra then offers some further insight. For example, Brad worked on healing his experience of sexual abuse in the lower chakras and then was drawn to the insight chakra:

> *...I can see that I was totally innocent. I was a kid. I have no responsibility for what happened. It is all on him (the abuser). I see this so clearly and I never saw it before, even though I have been told that many times. Now I get it. It is so clear I don't have to pay for that anymore. I am free of it.*

This was an important insight for Brad, as he and most victims of sexual abuse carry an unwarranted sense of responsibility for what happened to them. Brad could now completely let go and move on, for he could see it clearly for himself.

Sheryl looks forward to visiting her brother and his family but says that there is something dissatisfying about it and she usually comes back feeling depressed. After some discussion in which she tried to put her finger on what it was but couldn't, we did some Traya and she was led to the insight chakra:

---

19. *Merriam-Webster,* "Insight (2)," accessed January 1, 2016, http://www.merriam-webster.com/dictionary/insight.

...My spirit is crushed as they are really not interested in me.
...It feels so claustrophobic and thick—always at the mercy of their mood.

Then she had further insight:

...I don't belong to groups because of this. I didn't know all the places that I felt strangled.
...I feel strangled by people's vision of me from how I was in the past and not knowing how different I am now.

With this chakra, insights flow freely and are not always clearly tied to surfaced memories, nor is it always clear what negative energy to release. So one may not know what to do next as we always want to clear out negative energy samskaras when working with a chakra. My approach to deal with this is after the insight arises, ask what negative energy to let go out. For example, while writing this section I decided to work with it a little myself. I focused on the center of my forehead and asked for "any insight related to getting this book published" and what came was this:

...Stand in the lotus and let it grow up around you.

This was such a liberating insight. I took this to mean to just do it, and as this book nears completion, the energy will be there to take it where it needs to go—to do it with grounding, centeredness, and consciousness.

I could have left it there, but I know that there is usually an associated samskara so I asked, "What negative energy needs to be released?" and this came:

...All of the brainwashing around book publishing that we are inundated with. "Be sure you do this, or do that," etc.

My answer says that I don't have to do anything but what I am doing. Working on the book to the best of my ability.

It is appropriate that a secondary chakra such as the insight chakra would provide an answer related to the function of the one above it—

the crown chakra and its connection to both brainwashing and manifestation.

••• EXERCISE: TRAYA PRACTICE AT THE •••
THIRD EYE CHAKRA (AJNA)

Grounding

Ground by sitting up straight, focusing on the soles of your feet, and breathing in and out of the chakras at the soles of your feet.

Basic Technique

We will use the basic technique in which one deliberately picks a chakra to work with and the third eye chakra is focused on. Instead of just asking for memories, try this guided approach.

Start by grounding.

Step 1: Focus—Keep your attention at the point between your eyebrows and breathe in and out gently.

Step 2: Surface—Adopt the letting stance and ask, "What positive things about myself am I denying?" Wait until an answer appears. You receive something like, "You are smarter than you think." Now we must go one step further because it is a positive answer and ask, "What memories are here that contribute to my denying good things about myself?"

Step 3: Release—Note the memory and start to let negative energy go out by visualizing it coming out of the chakra. You can move to the next step or go back to step 2 and surface another memory adding to the chain of negative energy going out. After you are finished surfacing memories for this session, let all of the negative energy go out and wait until the outflow stops.

Step 4: Replace and Imprint—Visualize positive energy coming in (rays from the sun) and taking up the space that was taken up by the negative energy that went out. Ask, "What is this positive energy bringing in with it?" Note the words that appear in your mind.

Ground yourself again.

There is no scene from nature step here as the third eye chakra is beyond the physical realm and the five elements.

••• EXERCISE: TRAYA PRACTICE AT THE ••• INSIGHT CHAKRA (SATYAMANAS)

Let's use the basic technique again. You ground by breathing in and out of the soles of your feet.

Step 1: Focus—Keep your attention in the center of the forehead and breathe in and out gently.

Step 2: Surface—Adopt the letting stance and ask, "What memories are here?" Sometimes it is not clear what the negative aspect of the memory is here. If it is not clear ask, "What is the negative aspect of this memory?"

Step 3: Release—Note the memory and start to let negative energy go out by visualizing it coming out of the chakra. Keep surfacing memories and adding to the chain of negative energy going out or proceed to step 4.

Step 4: Replace and Imprint—Visualize positive energy coming in (rays from the sun) and taking up the space that was taken up by the negative energy that went out. Ask, "What is this positive energy bringing in with it?" Note the words that appear in your mind.

Ground.

There is no scene from nature step with the secondary chakras.

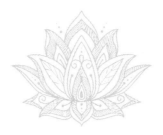

Chapter 12

THE CROWN CHAKRA (SAHASRARA)

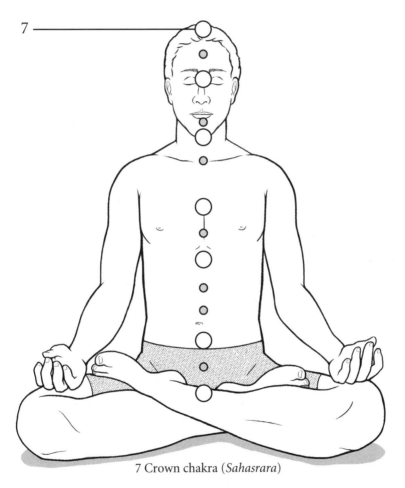

7 Crown chakra (*Sahasrara*)

Figure 12: Seventh Chakra

The Crown Chakra (Sahasrara)

- **Function:** autonomy
- **Attributes:** connection to the universe, spiritual maturity, manifestation, truth filter, liberation from false beliefs, wisdom, elevation, understanding, freedom, vision, power, influence, ebullience, bliss
- **Attribute paradox:** "I don't believe in myself."
- **Common issues in sahasrara:** attachment to false beliefs, easily influenced, follower

The crown chakra is referred to as the *mahapadma*, or great lotus. It is said to have twenty rows of fifty petals (one thousand total) all facing downward. In the yogic and Buddhist texts, large numbers such as one thousand or ten thousand are used to denote limitlessness. For example, in the Buddhist question, "The ten thousand things return to the one, where does the one return to?" the ten thousand things refer to everything—everything returns to the one.

Located at the crown of the head, the crown chakra is the culmination of the kundalini quest—the full bloom of the lotus—boundless consciousness. It is comprehension at a higher level than what is possible by the solar plexus mind tied to intellect and ego, for it connects directly to universal knowledge. Science can never fully comprehend the universe, as science is a solar plexus chakra construction and as such is limited, while the universe is limitless. The third eye chakra enables us to see clearly and the crown chakra provides an even more expanded perspective, spiritual knowledge, and autonomy. It connects us directly to sustenance from the spiritual source and when the crown chakra is strong and we are grounded in the root chakra, we can slip into *samadhi* (a deep meditative state) more readily.

The crown chakra is a truth filter, providing a reference point so that when indirect teachings, such as some of those passed down through the generations or that come from institutions, don't ring true, they are readily discarded. When beliefs are imposed, however, then samskaras form.

A major samskara here is that too much attention is given to the material world and not enough to the spiritual. Our society elevates materialism and we believe that if we acquire a lot then we will be happy. Religious, academic, and scientific authorities hold sway over our beliefs, and intuitive knowledge is demeaned and discounted. There are huge institutions and organizations all serving unconsciousness. Now we can see our collective insanity and understand that, in actuality, material things and attainments don't have that much to offer; and that is why people are always searching for more and more gratification. There is something within us that does not allow us to be happy unless we are connected spiritually. Its main purpose is to move us toward truth so that we can bloom fully. Just as the subtle body has been overlooked for so long, so it is within the subtle body— the crown chakra needs more attention from us.

Autonomy, Freedom, Liberation

When we work with the crown chakra, we enter the realm of autonomy. Autonomy means that we are free to think and act without yielding to influence from others. We realize that we can be social and connected and still be autonomous. The spiritual path is our own path for it is personal transformation that we seek. In the crown chakra, we realize that most samskaras are related to false beliefs imposed by familial, social, religious, and cultural indoctrinations.

Samskaric wounds appear early in life, when we are told what to believe instead of allowed to develop our own spiritual connections. It is not acknowledged that we have within us a connection to spirit that allows us to develop our own understanding of who we are and what we are doing here, but instead we are indoctrinated.

The crown chakra is the storehouse of our beliefs. One cannot comprehend the depth of the "programming" that we each experience in our cultures until one works with this energy and surfaces them one by one. These implanted falsehoods lie deep in our minds and we are often unaware of them—and even if aware, we don't understand the impact they have on our lives. Some are not so surprising—for myself and female clients that I work with, it often arises that "woman are considered second-class citizens" in all of the major religions. This samskara interferes with the growth and development of women both externally, in the religion itself, and internally, within the aspirant. In a book review of *The Hidden Lamp*, this point is addressed.

> Of course women practiced Zen in the old days. Of course, some were equals of the great male teachers. But for the most part these women and their stories were marginalized in the most prominent Chinese lineage charts and lamp records. These omissions have left women in the dark. It has denied them a place within the tradition, excluded them from authority and has suggested—not very subtly—that illumination was not for them—women could not serve as bearers of the lamp.[20]

Indeed, there are a lot of mixed messages in historical Buddhism. The Buddha accepted women as aspirants and stated that they could become enlightened. Yet, during different periods, devoted female aspirants, regardless of their attainment, were told that they must wait to be reborn a male in order to attain to full Buddhahood. A variety of different types of limitations are still imposed on women in modern religious society.

Limiting beliefs based on gender, race, religion, etc., impact everyone, not only the one belonging to the disparaged group, but the one harboring the beliefs also. Remember, these false beliefs are based on limiting samskaras in sahasrara suppressing its positive attributes. So both the discriminator and the discriminated are wounded as they both have the limiting samskaras. False beliefs are injurious, period. Whatever group is targeted feels diminished, takes in the false belief and has difficulty standing in their own power. The discriminating group is also diminished, although in more subtle ways. Any samskaras in the crown chakra bring with it diminishment, and the weakening of the connection to the higher source. Note also that prejudice

---

20. Barry Briggs, "Revision of 'The Hidden Lamp: Stories from Twenty Five Centuries of Awakened Women' by Florence Caplow and Susan Moon," *Primary Point*, Winter 2015, 18.

creates a wound in the heart chakra that contributes to a painful sense of disconnection—again for both parties.

False beliefs are everywhere and just seem to "float" out there in the ozone. We are always being influenced by our culture and are constantly picking up memes. Memes are "an idea, behavior, style, or usage that spreads from person to person within a culture."[21] These can then crystalize into beliefs and stereotypes.

With religion it goes both ways. We are indoctrinated into the religion we are born into and the opposite is true also:

> No religion exists in a vacuum. On the contrary, every faith is rooted in the soil in which it is planted. It is a fallacy to believe that people of faith derive their values primarily from their Scriptures. The opposite is true. People of faith insert their values into their Scriptures, reading them through the lens of their own cultural, ethnic, nationalistic and even political perspectives.[22]

We each have within the crown—and all of the chakras—a "truth monitor." We are wired to live in truth and every experience and belief is "reviewed" by this monitor. If negative or untruthful, a samskara appears. This can be challenging for those who have treasured their religious connections and hold dear certain beliefs. Working with Jim, who has a dedicated spiritual practice of meditation, the issue of religion came up here in the crown chakra:

> ... The religion I grew up with has a lot of negative press recently. I have always seen it as a duality, with mainly saintly, devoted people and a few selfish and evil people in the wrong jobs. What is coming through for me is: "That is not true."

21. *Merriam-Webster,* "Meme (1)," accessed January 1, 2016, http://www.merriam-webster.com/dictionary/meme.

22. Reza Aslan, "Bill Maher Isn't the Only One Who Misunderstands Religion," *New York Times*, October 8, 2014, editorial, https://www.nytimes.com/2014/10/09/opinion/bill-maher-isnt-the-only-one-who-misunderstands-religion.html.

Jim handled this knowledge well because he had already done a lot of Traya work and was not so dependent on outside forces—his locus of influence had already shifted to internal. (See chapter 5).

Another session with Jim surfaced the following:

> ...Everyone that I knew growing up was so oppressed by institutions. Everybody else had all the power and there was no standing up to them. The only hope was to someday get a job with one of them and then really lose your autonomy.

This is reminiscent of Foucault's position that "power somehow inheres in institutions themselves rather than in the individuals that make those institutions function."[23] Another samskara came up:

> ...Religion was imposed on me. I grew up in it and took in all those beliefs even though it didn't resonate with me. Rituals and pomp further inculcated their power and ownership of the truth.

Not just religious but all types of false beliefs are oppressive and limiting. Despite attempts to eradicate poverty and "lift up" the people trapped in it, poverty itself has a relentless way of continuing. Lotus grew up in a poor area. When working here, the following two issues came up:

> ...When you grow up in a ghetto, it is an unstated fact that you are involved in a dead end. Everyone assumes that you belong there and that is where you will stay. And everyone else belongs there too.
> ...It is also believed that there is nothing positive about the people there—they are defined by their poverty not their humanity.

These types of beliefs keep many people trapped in poverty.

Our beliefs about aging too can be hindrances. June was led to the crown chakra when we addressed the issue of finding productive activities in her life.

---

23. Dino Franco Felluga, *Critical Theory: The Key Concepts* (New York: Routledge, 2015), 238.

...I am too old and time is running out.

After we let the negative energy related to this belief out, these words came in with the positive:

...You are never too old and time never runs out.

I wonder just how much of the malaise and decrepitude of aging is a meme that is pervasive in our society. One study done with a group of elderly men when they lived for several weeks in an environment replicating their youth showed exactly that. They watched sports, television shows and listened to music from an era of their youth. They imagined themselves to be in that time again discussing current events of the time with each other. At the end of the study, "They were suppler, showed greater manual dexterity and sat taller. Perhaps most improbable, their sight improved. Independent judges said they looked younger." [24]

It is not only societal beliefs that imbed in the crown chakra and impede us, but personal ones also. I was working with a small group designed to help the members get a firm foothold on the Traya path. At the last session I had them focus on the crown and ask, "What negative beliefs are in my way?" This was the first time that they ever worked with this chakra. Following are some examples of what came immediately into their minds:

Ted:...*When I was six, my mother made fun of my being hairy. This made me believe that I am unattractive.*

Jess:...*My son is twenty-five and still dependent on me financially in some ways.*

He was annoyed with his son and wanted to change this pattern. He wanted his son to grow up and take responsibility for his life. While working here, he remembered how he always did things for him:

---

24. Bruce Grierson, "What If Age Were Nothing But a Mind-Set?" *New York Times,* October 22, 2014, MM52.

...I never believed in his ability to stand on his own feet, doing things for him since he was small.

Jess saw that he actually created this dynamic with his son, dropped his annoyance, and became determined to disconnect gently and give his son space to blossom on his own:

Zara: *...I was invited to the movies with a friend and her family and I wanted to go with them. My brother said he would come home from work early so that we could go and visit a relative that I liked. He didn't come home early and I missed out on the movie. The belief that I took in was to forgo what I want so as not to inconvenience others. I have been doing that my entire life.*

Marion: *...I was interested in art but felt that I couldn't follow that road because I was told that I would never be successful or be able to support myself. My parents lived in such limitation. They went to work in menial jobs and they came home. Their perspective was so limited and I picked that up from them.*

Spiritual Maturity, Liberation, Knowledge, and Understanding

We are turning our experiences over to the experts for analysis and interpretation when we can be doing that ourselves. The crown chakra tells us that the same is true of the spiritual path. We learn that not only have we been unconscious to so much but that everyone is unconscious to some extent—even many spiritual teachers. This chakra asks that we become our own guru and liberate ourselves from false beliefs. Only commit to a path because the spiritual truths of the teachings resonate with us and because of the *prajna* (wisdom) that arises, not because of outside influence, spiritual materialism or cultural bias. The Buddha advised us not to follow him blindly but to test the teachings out for ourselves and follow those that are true. Patanjali warns against domination of the *vrtti* of preconceived beliefs (no matter how authoritative) and tells us to be present in our experience. It is in the crown chakra that you become a spiritual "grown-up" and spiritually autonomous, because you have dropped the ego identity and have connected directly to a higher spiritual force. This doesn't mean that you cannot belong to a spiritual group or organization and practice with other people, it means that the responsibility is on you to determine what is true or not. The truth becomes our guru because we now have direct access to the limitless, all-encompassing, transcendental truth and wisdom.

Elevation

When the crown chakra is strong, then we are less likely to become wrapped up in or taken over by the solar plexus chakra's tendency for grasping and clinging. There is a sense of transcendence from worldly concerns while, at the same time, being fully engaged in the world. We understand what is really important and put our energies there.

Belief and the Body

The power of the mind to change biology is now taken for granted and scientists incorporate it into every clinical trial for new drugs and treatments. It is called the placebo effect.

Placebo—simply thinking you will get better can actually make you better. Patients experience positive effects from drugs merely because they expect to. Clinical-trial participants often report a wide variety of positive relief even when given sugar pills and told they were drugs.

Nocebo—simply thinking you will get worse can actually make you worse. Patients experience negative side effects from drugs merely because they expect to when told about side effects. These complaints may include burning sensations, vomiting, and even upper-respiratory-tract infections. Many participants reported these problems even when they were part of control groups that were taking a sugar pill.

It has even been shown that people with DID, or dissociative identity disorder (formerly known as multiple personality disorder), can have different physical problems depending on the identity they are manifesting:

"They may have different handedness, wear glasses with different prescriptions, and have allergies to different substances."[25] Entirely different physical states within the same body!

Even before we reached the crown chakra, our Traya work had already proved to us the power of the mind. We have seen how our minds created both intra- and interpersonal difficulties due to outside events and we also saw how our minds healed these same issues. We have also seen that certain emotional states are associated with corresponding changes in brain chemistry. For example, depressed states show correlated changes in brain chemistry that antidepressant medications are designed to correct. This has led to the false belief that chemistry is what is causing the depression when it is actually the reverse—the depression (a very samskaric heart chakra) is causing the changes in brain chemistry. We know this because when we heal the heart chakra completely with Traya, the brain chemistry adjusts accordingly and there is no longer a need for these medications. We are awed at how powerful our minds are.

Manifestation, Power, and Influence

I was surprised to find that manifestation in this world is such an important function of this chakra, as I expected it to be more concerned with transcendence. The crown chakra tells us that we must create the world that we need in order to thrive, and this is done through this energy. We find that we are beings with a power that we didn't know that we had—not the will-oriented *making* of the solar plexus chakra but the manifesting of our heart's desires. A mistaken belief that most of us hold is that power lies outside of us, when in actuality the reverse is true.

It is through the crown chakra that universal consciousness comes into the level of form. Physics shows that energy creates matter and the shorter the wavelength, the more energy, and thus more power. The crown chakra's energy has the shortest wavelength of any chakra

25. Gerald C. Davison and John M. Neale, *Abnormal Psychology* (New York: John Wiley and Sons, 1998), 170.

and is thus the most powerful. While every chakra has an impact on the outside world and creates situations in the outside world based on its health status, the crown manifests desires, vision, and purpose in life via its connection to the creative power of the universe. It is through this energy that our higher good manifests and our dreams come true. Our deepest desires come into fruition as long as they are aligned with spiritual growth and direction and the good of others. In Hinduism there is the "wish-fulfilling cow" *Kamadhenu* that is believed to become accessible in this chakra. She is the divine mother of all cows and represents the creative manifestation energy of the crown chakra.

In order to manifest, we must have a vision. Before we change the world, we must have a vision for our own lives and what needs to come next. Our vision manifests from our heart's desire not from our willpower—*if* we maintain a strong moment connection. The moment is the place of manifestation. The creative energy of the crown chakra will only manifest if the moment connection and the connection between the two lotus poles, the root chakra (muladhara) and the crown chakra (sahasrara), are strong. When you heal these two chakras and also maintain a strong moment connection, you unleash the energy of manifestation.

Self-actualization is only one of the benefits achieved here. We realize also that our purpose is not to escape this life or to escape to some heaven. Since we are all connected, there can be no heaven while others are suffering on earth. As we work with the higher chakras, our perspective shifts. We realize that the world is not here for us to exploit but we are here for the world. Our job is not only to align with the creative power of the universe but to actually manifest something in the world—to influence this world in some helpful way. I once heard a Zen master say, "Enlightenment is believing in yourself 100 percent." When you believe in yourself, then you have influence and power.

The crown chakra takes time to get to know. We need to spend time here, and the work that we do to arrive here is well worth the effort. We do this by healing the lower chakras and meditating as much as possible, as it is most fully activated when we meditate. Spiritual power and knowledge then dominate our consciousness rather than the distractions of the material world.

When we connect with a healthy crown chakra in meditation, we experience bliss. Being on a spiritual path means being on a path of energy aligned with truth, and it means doing the practices on that path and understanding how the truth functions in us for the good of all.

••• EXERCISE: TRAYA PRACTICE AT THE ••• CROWN CHAKRA (SAHASRARA)

Grounding

Ground by sitting up straight, focusing on the soles of your feet, and breathing in and out of the chakras at the soles of your feet.

Basic Technique

It is best to wait until the lower chakras have been strengthened before working here. Rarely will you be led here by any of the deep mind–directed techniques for surfacing samskaras until then. So that you can get a sense of this energy, we are going to use a variation of the basic technique in that we will focus on the chakra, but instead of starting by asking for memories, we are going to first ask for false beliefs. This is a very subtle energy and it may be difficult for the beginner to tune in here and surface a memory. This will help.

> **Step 1: Focus**—Keep your attention at the crown of your head and breathe in and out gently.
>
> **Step 2: Surface**—Breathe in and out gently and ask, "What false beliefs are here and where did they come from?" After something comes into your mind, you can ask, "What else?" or move on to step 3.
>
> **Step 3: Release**—Note the belief and associated memory or memories. Let negative energy go out by visualizing it coming out of the chakra, waiting until the outflow stops.
>
> **Step 4: Replace and Imprint**—Visualize positive energy coming in (rays from the sun) and taking up the space that was taken up

by the negative energy that went out. Ask, "What is this positive energy bringing in with it?" Note the words that appear in your mind.

There is no scene from nature here as sahasrara is beyond the realm of elements.

Ground yourself back in your body by breathing in and out of the soles of your feet.

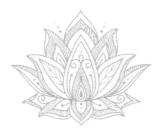

CONCLUSION

I have presented a lot of information in this book. I want to reiterate that you do not have to know anything in order to successfully use the Traya techniques presented here. Many years ago, when I first thought about writing a book on this topic, I thought, "How will I make an entire book out of such a simple technique?" Like the Traya process itself, over the years it grew up around me. That is the point that I would like to leave you with. Keep it simple and just let it grow up through you and around you. Take the same approach that you would take with meditation and yoga—it is the practice itself that counts, and over time it works its magic on you. You only need to show up.

Not everyone is spiritually inclined. If you have read this book, you are one of those so inclined. While it is a great privilege to be spiritually aware, this precious instinct also comes with responsibility. The responsibility to answer the question, "Why am I here?" Then you can use your influence to heal the world in your own unique way. Now that we know how truly sensitive we all are, we must put energy into cultivating our hearts and use our interactions with others in a healing way. Connecting with everyday experience right now, moment by moment, we can use that experience to feed our blooming Lotus of Full Potential. Like the lotus, our job is to produce something beautiful—our true selves reflected in the physical world.

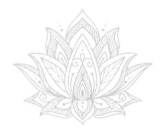

GLOSSARY

Abhaya Chakra: Secondary chakra located about one inch above the pelvic chakra (svadhisthana). Its function is being unafraid of the power of others.

Ahimsa: Nonviolence.

Ajna Chakra: Third eye chakra. Primary chakra located between the eyebrows. Main function is clear perception.

Akasha: Subtle ethereal energy.

Anahata Chakra: Heart chakra. Primary chakra located in the center of the chest. Main function is connection to self, others, nature, life, and spirit.

Atiloka Chakra: Imagination chakra. Secondary chakra located between the root (muladhara) and pelvic (svadhisthana) chakras. Function is imagination.

Attribute Paradox: Attribute of a chakra is samskaric and contradicts the chakra's function.

Authentic Self: Self that is readily apparent when the mind is free of the pain body.

Bijas: Seed sounds that stimulate a chakra.

Chakras: Subtle energy centers in the body determining various states of mind, the mind–body connection, and influencing the health of the body.

Dantian: Chinese term for svadhisthana, the pelvic chakra.

Deep Mind: One of the two minds (surface is the other). Resonates with the truth and actively attempts to communicate it to us.

Diagnostic Scene: Image that arises in step 5 of Traya Practice containing elements from nature that appear when concentrating attention at one of the lower five primary chakras. Can be used to determine relative health of a chakra.

Empty Opulence: There is plenty of money and status but a significant lack of the connection energy that one really needs—produces a sense of emptiness in the heart.

Hungry Ghosts: Beings with long thin necks representing the afflictive state of a grasping, greedy mind in Buddhism.

Ida Nadi: Lunar nadi originating in the root chakra and spiraling up around the central sushumna channel and coming out of the left nostril.

Inner Compass: Three chakras that help us navigate through life indicating when we are going in the right or wrong direction—heart (anahata), solar plexus (manipura), and third eye (ajna) chakras.

Inner Eye: Images appear in the mind when focus of attention is on the subtle body via the Inner Eye.

Inner Teacher: Messenger from higher mind that guides us with direction and advice in the form of insights and positive imprints in the Traya process—also while meditating.

Inner Voice: Information is given to us through words that appear in the mind when working with Traya; e.g., surfaced samskaras, positive imprints, guidance, etc.

Inside/Outside Maxim: Proposition that what is inside the mind is manifested in the outside world. Both positive and negative energy in the subtle body attracts situations that reflect it.

Introjection: The taking in of subtle energy from others and from the environment (pick-ups).

Kamadhenu: "Wish-fulfilling cow." Hindu deity associated with the crown chakra (sahasrara).

Klesas: Destructive emotions such as anger and fear and other mind afflictions such as jealousy, distrust, greed, etc. Three klesas of ignorance, attachment, and aversion, also known as the three poisons in Buddhism.

Kundalini Shakti: Spiritual energy lying dormant in the root chakra. Meditation, pranayama, yoga, and mantras are practices designed to awaken it and have it rise up to the sahasrara or crown chakra.

Lego Effect: Samskaras resulting from actions taken due to previous samskaras that build a vasana.

Locus of Influence: Where one looks for guidance. With weak inner resources before Traya healing, one looks to others. With strong inner resources, one looks within.

Lotus Energy: Spiritual prana.

Lotus of Full Potential: The Inner Lotus in full bloom. Flowering of the authentic self. Leads to the attainment of one's true purpose in life.

Lotus Poles: Root chakra (muladhara) facing up and crown (sahasrara) chakra facing down. Kundalini originates in root and moves up to crown while, at the same time, maintaining a strong root connection.

Mahapadma: Sanskrit for "Great Lotus" refers to the crown chakra with 1,000 petals.

Manifestation Chakras: The crown chakra (sahasrara), the heart chakra (anahata), and the root chakra (muladhara). These energies combine vision, desire, and action leading to manifestation.

Manipura Chakra: Solar plexus chakra located at the diaphragm. Function is the I-consciousness.

Manipurism: Statement or behavior indicating the domination of, and over identification with, manipura—the solar plexus chakra.

Mantra: Sanskrit term defined as a "mystical verse or charm." Sanskrit mantras contain sounds designed to activate the chakras and stimulate latent spiritual energy.

Mudra: Specific gesture or pose that affects the flow of prana in the body.

Mukta: Secondary chakra located between the solar plexus chakra (manipura) and abhaya chakra (fearless). Function is "letting go."

Muladhara Chakra: Root chakra located at the base of the spine. Main function is safety and security in physical environment.

Nadi(s): Subtle energy pathways throughout the human body.

Noble Eightfold Path: Fourth of the Four Noble Truths outlined by the Buddha offered as the way out of suffering: Right View, Right Intention, Right Speech, Right Action, Right Livelihood, Right Effort, Right Mindfulness, Right Concentration.

Om/Lam: Bija sounds of the crown chakra (sahasrara) and the root chakra (muladhara) connecting the two lotus poles. Use to assist in meditation.

Padmasana: Seated cross-legged asana. Lotus pose. Meditation mudra.

Pain Body: Collection of negative samskaras and vasanas that produce painful thoughts and feelings and move one toward unhealthy behaviors while also attracting negativity.

Pancha Mahabhutas: Five great elements—ether, air, fire, water, earth.

Patanjali: Indian compiler of the *Yoga Sutras* circa 200 CE.

Pick-ups: Introjection of others' energy dynamics into our own due to repeated exposure when growing up.

Pingala Nadi: Solar nadi spiraling around the central sushumna channel that comes out the right nostril.

Positive Imprint: Positive words given by the higher mind in step 4 of the Traya technique.

Prajna: Highest form of wisdom.

Prana: Subtle life energy that flows throughout and animates the mind, body, and the entire universe. Five types govern the function of the human mind and body: prana, samana, apana, vyana, and udana.

Pranayama: Yogic breathing practices designed to move prana within the body.

Pranothana: Positive charge of new energy into the subtle body during the Traya practice stimulating the subtle body.

Rajas: One of the three gunas—active energy.

Sahasrara Chakra: Crown chakra located at the top of the head. Function is autonomy.

Samadhi: Deep meditative state.

Samskaras: Memory imprints that leave an energetic residue in one or more chakras. Negative are mind toxins—positive are mind nourishment.

Sattva: One of the three gunas—subtle, calm, and peaceful.

Satyahridaya: Asking chakra. Secondary chakra located at the collarbone between the heart (anahata) and throat (vishuddha) chakras. Function is asking for what is in the heart.

Satyamanas: True speech chakra. Secondary chakra located at the top of the neck between the throat (vishuddha) and the third eye (ajna) chakras. Function is speaking the truth.

Satyavadya: Insight chakra. Secondary chakra located at the center of the forehead. Function is insight.

Secondary Chakras: Seven small chakras located between the seven primary chakras—atiloka (imagination); abhaya (fearlessness); mukta (letting go); vajrahridaya (self-esteem); satyahridaya (asking for what is in the heart); satyamanas (speaking the truth); and satyavadya (insight).

Shakti: Spiritual feminine energy.

Subtle Body: Energy body within the physical body composed of chakras and nadis through which prana flows.

Sukhasana: Easy pose. Cross-legged alternative to full lotus pose in meditation.

Surface Mind: Conscious mind.

Sushumna Nadi: Central nadi runs from base of spine in the root chakra (muladhara) up to sahasrara the crown chakra.

Svadhisthana: Pelvic chakra. Located one inch below the navel. Main function is personal power in relationships.

Tamas: One of the three gunas—heavy, inertia.

Tantra: Indian beliefs and practices that explore the relationship between divine energy (macrocosm) and the person (microcosm).

Tao: Chinese religion or philosophy that proposes living in harmony with the Way (Tao).

Ten Directions: North, south, east, west, northwest, northeast, southwest, southeast, up, and down.

Three Gunas: Sattva (light, consciousness), rajas (active), and tamas (heavy, dark); qualities in both material world and human consciousness.

True Body: Positive state with minimal or no samskaric pain body.

Truth factor: Traya concept that proposes that the human psyche is attuned to and aligned with truth.

Vajrahridaya: Self-esteem chakra. Secondary chakra located at lower sternum between the solar plexus and heart chakras. Function is self-esteem.

Vasana: String of similarly themed samskaras.

Veil of Unawareness: Allows the surface mind to operate without being overwhelmed by input from the deep mind. Barrier between what is "in the mind versus what is on the mind."

Vishuddha Chakra: Throat chakra located in the center of the neck. Function is self-expression.

Vritti: Sanskrit term meaning waves or turbulence.

Yukta Triveni: "Three streams." Three major nadis—sushumna, ida, and pingala.

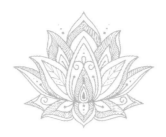

ACKNOWLEDGMENTS

I am forever indebted to Nancy Rosanoff for starting me on this incredible journey. Special gratitude to my two intrepid main readers, Clare Ellis and Nina Levenson, for their efforts and insights. To my writing buddy Shizuka Otake for lightening up this process with fun times out of town and Preston Browning of Wellspring House for providing personal encouragement along with a nourishing country setting for writers. The Writers Room in NYC contributed the city version. To Marty Epstein for his freely given Sanskrit expertise and my colleagues Betsy Spiegle and Ann Burke for their enthusiastic encouragement. I am grateful for all of my friends and family who believed in me and encouraged me along the way, especially my daughter Kristen, who really gets it. Thanks to Angela Wix and Brian Erdrich at Llewellyn for their professionalism, editing thoroughness, and patience. I am grateful to Michael Larsen for his ideas regarding the initial direction and structure of this book and to Celeste Mendelsohn for her insights regarding the application of Traya to yoga therapy. To Scott and Jamie Harig, my new yoga teachers, for their dedication, expertise, and especially warmth over the past year. Special thanks to everyone who has worked with me doing the actual Traya work and particularly those whose material appears in this book—it is your courage and openness in sharing your inner world so fully, your hard work and generosity, that has made this book possible.

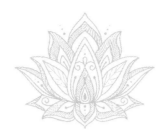

INDEX

Thoughts, 2, 3, 10, 12, 13, 15–17, 19, 39, 40, 44, 54, 60, 62, 64, 76, 77, 94, 98, 101, 102, 107, 121, 130, 131, 133, 136–138, 172, 177, 180, 185, 198, 228
Throat chakra, 5, 22, 31, 35, 45, 54, 67, 76, 77, 81, 87, 92, 105, 107, 144, 175–183, 185–188, 190–192, 200, 230
Time, 2–5, 10–12, 15, 16, 20, 28, 32, 36, 40, 44, 47, 49, 51, 54, 55, 62, 75, 78, 79, 81–83, 86, 89, 93, 95, 97–103, 105, 108, 111, 114, 116, 121, 123, 130, 132–134, 138, 139, 142–145, 156, 158, 161, 163, 168, 173, 179–182, 184, 185, 187, 188, 196–198, 200, 214, 215, 217, 219, 223, 227
Transcendence, 217, 218
Transition, 21, 83
Transformation, 1, 7, 53, 75, 92, 94, 103, 211
Trauma, 123, 134, 198
True nature, 93, 131
True speech chakra, 22, 30, 54, 175, 190, 191, 193, 229
Truth, 2, 11, 13, 15, 16, 27, 28, 30, 33, 37, 39, 46, 53, 54, 76, 94, 98, 139, 154, 162, 163, 167, 169, 189, 190, 193, 196–198, 200, 202–204, 210, 211, 213, 214, 217, 220, 226, 229, 230
Transcendental, 217
Trust, 4, 28, 53, 76, 81–83, 86, 96, 107, 111, 135, 138, 139, 142, 149, 154, 155, 157–160, 163, 167, 171, 201

Udana prana, 26, 46, 228
Unconscious, 9, 10, 57, 111, 178, 197, 216
Understanding, 5, 7, 27, 33, 55, 57, 58, 97, 105, 154, 155, 161, 167, 169, 196, 197, 210, 211, 216, 220
Undeserving, 169
Unimportant, 42, 124, 170
Universe, 3, 4, 27, 33, 80, 82, 87, 89, 96, 132, 154, 160, 162, 164, 203, 210, 219, 228
Uninteresting, 170

To Write to the Author

If you wish to contact the author or would like more information about book, please write to the author in care of Llewellyn Worldwide Ltd. and we will forward your request. Both the author and publisher appreciate hearing from you and learning of your enjoyment of this book and how it has helped you. Llewellyn Worldwide Ltd. cannot guarantee that every letter written to the author can be answered, but all will be forwarded. Please write to:

Trish O'Sullivan
℅ Llewellyn Worldwide
2143 Wooddale Drive
Woodbury, MN 55125-2989

Please enclose a self-addressed stamped envelope for reply,
or $1.00 to cover costs. If outside the U.S.A., enclose
an international postal reply coupon.

Many of Llewellyn's authors have websites with additional information and resources. For more information, please visit our website at http://www.llewellyn.com

GET MORE AT LLEWELLYN.COM

Visit us online to browse hundreds of our books and decks, plus sign up to receive our e-newsletters and exclusive online offers.

- **Free tarot readings** • **Spell-a-Day** • **Moon phases**
- **Recipes, spells, and tips** • **Blogs** • **Encyclopedia**
- **Author interviews, articles, and upcoming events**

GET SOCIAL WITH LLEWELLYN

Find us on 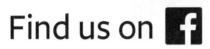 @LlewellynBooks
www.Facebook.com/LlewellynBooks

GET BOOKS AT LLEWELLYN

LLEWELLYN ORDERING INFORMATION

Order online: Visit our website at www.llewellyn.com to select your books and place an order on our secure server.

Order by phone:
- Call toll free within the US at 1-877-NEW-WRLD (1-877-639-9753)
- We accept VISA, MasterCard, American Express, and Discover.
- Canadian customers must use credit cards.

Order by mail:
Send the full price of your order (MN residents add 6.875% sales tax) in US funds plus postage and handling to: Llewellyn Worldwide, 2143 Wooddale Drive, Woodbury, MN 55125-2989

POSTAGE AND HANDLING

STANDARD (US):
(Please allow 12 business days)
$30.00 and under, add $6.00.
$30.01 and over, FREE SHIPPING.

INTERNATIONAL ORDERS,
INCLUDING CANADA:
$16.00 for one book, plus $3.00 for each additional book.

Visit us online for more shipping options. Prices subject to change.

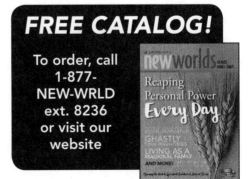

FREE CATALOG!

To order, call
1-877-
NEW-WRLD
ext. 8236
or visit our
website

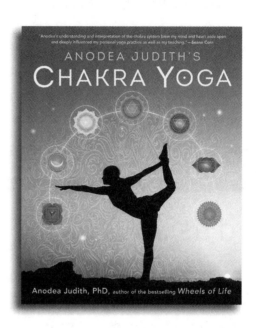

"Anodea's understanding and interpretation of the chakra system blew my mind and heart wide open and deeply influenced my personal yoga practice as well as my teaching." —Seane Corn

ANODEA JUDITH'S

CHAKRA YOGA

Anodea Judith, PhD, author of the bestselling *Wheels of Life*

Anodea Judith's Chakra Yoga
ANODEA JUDITH, PHD

As the architecture of the soul, the chakra system is the yoke of yoga—the means whereby mind and body, heaven and earth, and spirit and matter are joined together in the divine union that is the true meaning of yoga.

In this long-awaited book by acclaimed chakra expert Anodea Judith, you will learn how to use yoga's principles and practices to awaken the subtle body of energy and connect with your highest source. Using seven vital keys to unlock your inner temple, you will be guided through practices that open and activate each chakra through postures, bioenergetic exercises, breathing practices, mantras, guided meditation, and yoga philosophy. With beautiful step-by-step photographs for each of the poses, along with guidelines for deeper alignment and activation of the energy body, this book is a valuable resource for teachers and students alike.

978-0-7387-4444-5, 480 pp., 7½ x 9¼   **$27.99**

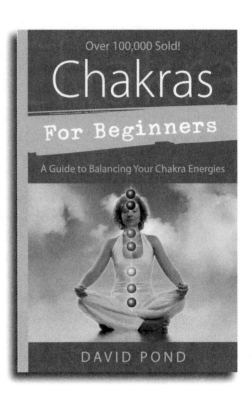

Over 100,000 Sold!

Chakras

For Beginners

A Guide to Balancing Your Chakra Energies

DAVID POND

Chakras for Beginners
A Guide to Balancing Your Chakra Energies
DAVID POND

You may think that difficult situations and emotions you experience are caused by other people or random events. This book will convince you that inner imbalance is not caused by situations in the outer world—instead, your imbalances create the situations that interfere with your sense of well-being and peace.

Chakras for Beginners explains how to align your energy on many levels to achieve balance and health from the inside out. In everyday terms, you will learn the function of the seven body-spirit energy vortexes called chakras. Practical exercises, meditations, and powerful techniques for working with your energy flow will help you overcome imbalances that block your spiritual progress.

- Discover colors and crystals that activate each chakra.
- Explore the balanced and unbalanced expressions of each chakra's energies: survival, sexuality, power, love, creativity, intuition, and spirituality.
- Practice spiritual exercises, visualizations, and meditations that bring your energies into balance.

978-1-56718-537-9, 192 pp., 5 ³⁄₁₆ x 8 $13.99

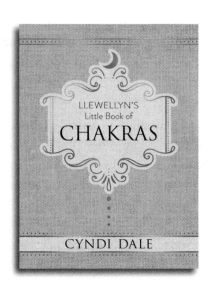

Llewellyn's Little Book of Chakras
Cyndi Dale

Chakras are subtle energy centers that affect all levels of your being: physical, psychological, and spiritual. In this pocket-size hardcover guide, you'll discover why these spinning wheels of energy are the key to living at your highest potential, with tips for using chakras to:

- Heal from physical and psychological wounds
- Express feelings easily and productively
- Transform work into a joyful vocation
- Solve financial and career difficulties
- Free repressed emotions
- Deal with life's puzzles and predicaments
- Soothe the heart and create more loving relationships

978-0-7387-5155-9, 240 pp., 4.63 x 6.25　　　　　　　　**$12.99**

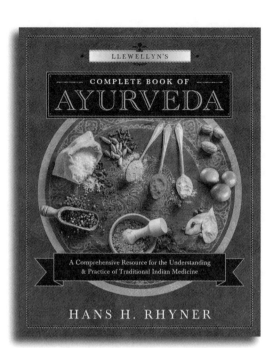

Llewellyn's Complete Book of Ayurveda
A Comprehensive Resource for the Understanding
& Practice of Traditional Indian Medicine
HANS H. RHYNER

Ayurveda is the art of good life and gentle healing. It is a holistic system of medicine that includes prevention, psychology, diet, and treatment. Join Hans H. Rhyner, a leading authority on Ayurveda, as he explores the principles, therapies, and collected knowledge of this powerful approach to health and well-being, including:

Anatomical Aspects (*Rachana Sharira*) • Evolutionary Physiology (*Kriya Sharira*) • Constitution (*Prakruti*) • Pathology (*Samprapti*) • Diagnostics (*Nidana*) • Pharmacology (*Dravya Guna*) • Treatment Strategies (*Chikitsa*) • Nutritional Sciences (*Annavijnana*) • Preventative Medicine (*Swasthavritta*) • Quintet of Therapeutics (Panchakarma) • Clinical Applications

978-0-7387-4868-9, 672 pp., 8 x 10   **$34.99**

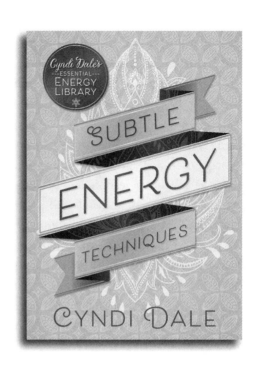

SUBTLE

ENERGY

TECHNIQUES

CYNDI DALE

Subtle Energy Techniques
Cyndi Dale

Renowned author Cyndi Dale invites you into the world of subtle energy, where you'll explore auras, chakras, intuition, and the basics of her groundbreaking energy techniques. Whether your goals are physical, psychological, or spiritual, these methods can help you achieve your desires, heal your wounds, and live an enlightened life.

978-0-7387-5161-0, 288 pp., 5 x 7   **$14.99**

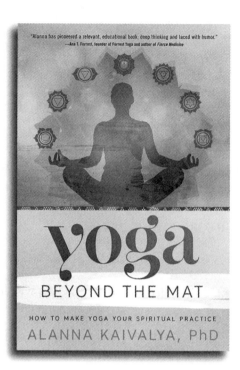

yoga

BEYOND THE MAT

HOW TO MAKE YOGA YOUR SPIRITUAL PRACTICE

ALANNA KAIVALYA, PhD

Yoga Beyond the Mat
How to Make Yoga Your Spiritual Practice
ALANNA KAIVALYA, PHD

While many engage in asana, the physical practice, yoga's most transformative effects are found in the realms of the spiritual and psychological. *Yoga Beyond the Mat* shows you how to develop a personal, holistic yoga practice to achieve lasting and permanent transformation. Join Alanna Kaivalya as she guides you through a complete range of topics, including:

- Removing Obstacles
- Appreciating the Present Moment
- Balancing the Chakras
- Healing Childhood Wounds
- Creating Your Own Rituals
- Transforming Your Archetypal Energy
- Entering the Blissful State

This book shows you that yoga doesn't make your life easier; it makes you better at your life. Through ritual, meditation, journaling, asana, and other spiritual practices, *Yoga Beyond the Mat* provides techniques for developing a personal mythology and allowing the ego to rest, leading modern-day yogis toward what they have been missing: the realization of personal bliss.

978-0-7387-4764-4, 264 pp., 6 x 9   **$16.99**

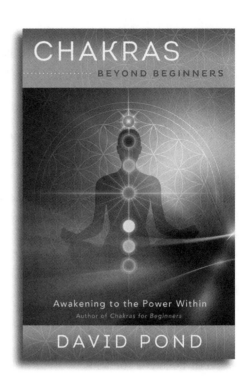

CHAKRAS
BEYOND BEGINNERS

Awakening to the Power Within
Author of *Chakras for Beginners*

DAVID POND

Chakras Beyond Beginners
Awakening to the Power Within
DAVID POND

Discover the path to your energetic core and bring each chakra into its full potential with *Chakras Beyond Beginners*. Building on concepts presented in *Chakras for Beginners*, David Pond takes you past basic understanding to explore the many ways chakras can enhance the flow of vital energy in all aspects of your life.

Learn how to identify and remove the obstacles that inhibit your energy, as well as how to keep that flow open. Raise your awareness of other people's energy fields and use it to improve your relationships. Find fulfillment, security, and happiness by balancing your chakras. With this guide, you'll unlock your true essence and the source of your well-being.

978-0-7387-4859-7, 240 pp., 5¼ x 8   **$16.99**

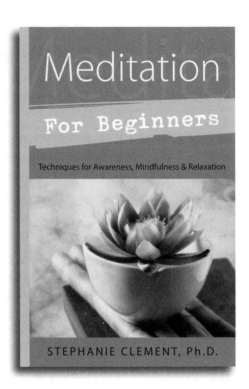

Meditation

For Beginners

Techniques for Awareness, Mindfulness & Relaxation

STEPHANIE CLEMENT, Ph.D.

Meditation for Beginners
Techniques for Awareness, Mindfulness & Relaxation
STEPHANIE CLEMENT

Break the barrier between your conscious and unconscious minds.

Perhaps the greatest boundary we set for ourselves is the one between the conscious and less conscious parts of our own minds. We all need a way to gain deeper understanding of what goes on inside our minds when we are awake, asleep, or just not paying attention. Meditation is one way to pay attention long enough to find out.

Meditation for Beginners offers a step-by-step approach to meditation, with exercises that introduce you to the rich possibilities of this age-old spiritual practice. Improve concentration, relax your body quickly and easily, work with your natural healing ability, and enhance performance in sports and other activities. Just a few minutes each day is all that's needed.

- Contains step-by-step meditation exercises.
- Shows how to develop a consistent meditation effort in just a few minutes each day.
- Explores many different ways to meditate, including kundalini yoga, walking meditation, dream meditation, tarot meditations, healing meditation.

978-0-7387-0203-2, 264 pp., 5³⁄₁₆ x 8   **$14.99**

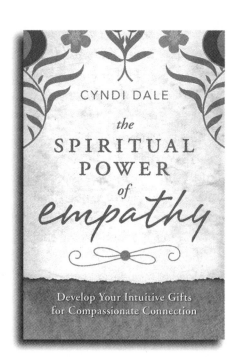

CYNDI DALE

the
SPIRITUAL
POWER
of
empathy

Develop Your Intuitive Gifts
for Compassionate Connection

The Spiritual Power of Empathy
Develop Your Intuitive Gifts for Compassionate Connection
CYNDI DALE

For some the empathic gift provides insight and inspiration, but for others empathy creates feelings of confusion and panic. *The Spiritual Power of Empathy* is a hands-on training course for empaths, showing you how to comfortably use this often-unrecognized ability for better relationships, career advancement, raising children, and healing the self and others.

Join popular author Cyndi Dale as she shares ways to develop the six empathic types, techniques for screening and filtering information, and tips for opening up to a new world of deeper connections with the loved ones in your life. Also includes important information for dealing with the difficulties empaths often face, such as being overwhelmed in a crowd.

978-0-7387-3799-7, 264 pp., 6 x 9   **$16.99**